SELF-ASSESSMENT GUIDE

to accompany

Respiratory Care
Principles & Practice

SELF-ASSESSMENT GUIDE

to accompany

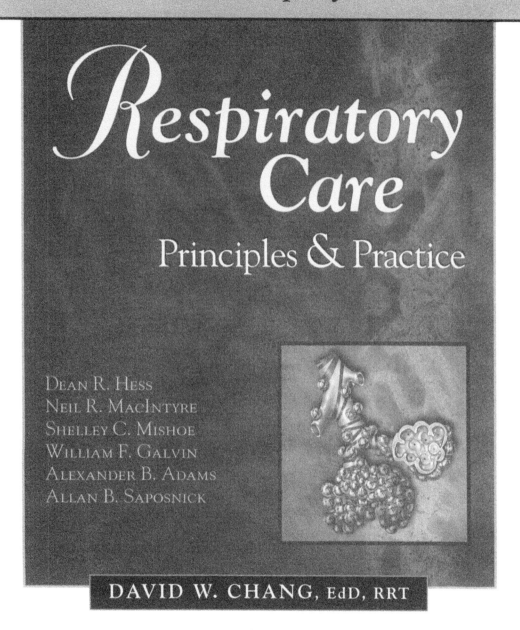

Respiratory
Care

Principles & Practice

DEAN R. HESS
NEIL R. MACINTYRE
SHELLEY C. MISHOE
WILLIAM F. GALVIN
ALEXANDER B. ADAMS
ALLAN B. SAPOSNICK

DAVID W. CHANG, EdD, RRT

Director of Clinical Education
Respiratory Therapy
Athens Technical College
Athens, Georgia

W.B. SAUNDERS COMPANY
Philadelphia London New York St. Louis Sydney Toronto

W.B. Saunders Company

The Curtis Center
Independence Square West
Philadelphia, Pennsylvania 19106

Acquisitions Editor: Karen Fabiano
Developmental Editor: Mindy Copeland
Project Manager: Gayle Morris
Cover Designer: Julia Dummitt

SELF-ASSESSMENT GUIDE TO ACCOMPANY
RESPIRATORY CARE: PRINCIPLES & PRACTICE

ISBN 0-7216-9696-1

Transferred to Digital Printing 2009

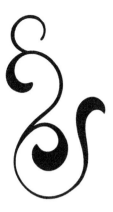

Preface

Research studies have shown that learning is more likely to occur when there is active participation by learners. Active learning takes place when the materials presented are pertinent and when immediate feedback is provided to the learners. The goal of this self-assessment study guide is to promote self-learning through the use of more than 1,700 multiple-choice questions that coincide with the learning objectives and other essential concepts of *Respiratory Care: Principles & Practice.*

Users of this self-assessment study guide should read all of the material in each chapter of the textbook and then complete the self-assessment questions in this study guide. Answer keys at the end of this study guide should be used to verify correct responses and to further review the material in the textbook. The minimum passing level for the questions in each chapter is set at 70%. This percentage can be calculated by dividing the number of correct answers by the total number of questions in each chapter. Users are encouraged to review the material in the textbook and repeat the self-assessment questions as often as necessary to master the content.

David W. Chang

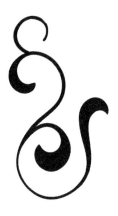

Acknowledgements

My gratitude goes to Dean Hess, the lead editor of *Respiratory Care: Principles & Practice*, for his trust in me by giving me the latitude to develop a study guide using a "self-assessment" format. I believe this format will serve the learners well in the process of active learning. Throughout the writing and editing stage of this study guide, the editorial and production team members of Harcourt Health Sciences made my task simple and enjoyable. They are Karen Fabiano, acquisitions editor, Mindy Copeland, developmental editor, Ellen Wurm, editorial assistant, and Jeanne Genz, production editor. I would like to express my sincere appreciation to my friend and colleague Art Jones for his careful review of the entire manuscript. His experience in respiratory care and education enhances the accuracy and clarity of this study guide. A special thank you is extended to Larry Carlisle, clinical manager of respiratory therapy at Athens Regional Hospital, for his help in clarifying selected areas in the study guide. It has always been a pleasure to work with Art and Larry on any project.

David W. Chang

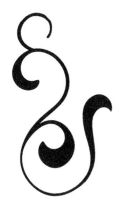

Contents

SELF-ASSESSMENT GUIDE

to accompany

Respiratory Care
Principles & Practice

CHAPTER 1

History of the Respiratory Care Profession

1. In the 1930s, _____ led to the use of _____ ventilators (iron lungs), considered one of the most significant technologic advances in the early days of respiratory care.
   A. tuberculosis; negative-pressure tank
   B. poliomyelitis; negative-pressure tank
   C. AIDS; positive-pressure
   D. Black Death; positive-pressure

2. In 1895, Karl von Linde was credited for the manufacturing of inexpensive _____ by using fractional distillation of liquefied air in the production of nitrogen.
   A. carbon dioxide
   B. helium
   C. carbon monoxide
   D. oxygen

3. Oxygen demand valves, WWII combat aviators, and high-altitude hypoxia contributed to the development and practical application of:
   A. intermittent positive pressure breathing (IPPB) devices.
   B. small volume nebulizers.
   C. oxygen masks.
   D. "iron lung" ventilator.

4. Dr. Levine organized the first training program for _____ as part of a department of chest diseases in Chicago's Michael Reese Hospital.
   A. respiratory therapists
   B. oxygen orderlies
   C. inhalation therapists
   D. certified respiratory therapists (CRTs) and registered respiratory therapists (RRTs)

5. The Inhalation Therapy Association (ITA), incorporated in Illinois in 1947, is now the:
   A. National Board for Respiratory Care (NBRC).
   B. American Association for Respiratory Care (AARC).
   C. American Respiratory Care Foundation (ARCF).
   D. Board of Medical Advisors (BOMA).

6. The first Conference on the Scientific Basis of Respiratory Therapy was held in 1974 at Sugarloaf, Philadelphia and the results led to the use of other respiratory care modalities in place of:
   A. IPPB.
   B. mechanical ventilation.
   C. blood gases.
   D. oxygen therapy.

7. Activities to gain licensure for respiratory therapists were started in _____. By mid-1999, licensure, certification, and registration laws are in effect in more than _____ states, the District of Columbia, and Puerto Rico.
   A. 1960, 20
   B. 1980, 20
   C. 1960, 40
   D. 1980, 40

8. CRCE are the education units for _____ and are _____ by most states for licensure.
   A. core respiratory care; required
   B. core respiratory care; not required
   C. continuing respiratory care; required
   D. continuing respiratory care; not required

9. The accreditation agency for respiratory care education programs is:
   A. RCAB.
   B. CoARC.
   C. JRCRTE.
   D. NBRC.

10. The credentialing agency for respiratory therapists is:
    A. ARCF.
    B. AARC.
    C. NBRC.
    D. CoARC.

11. All of the following are credentials awarded by the National Board for Respiratory Care *except*:
    A. RRT.
    B. RPFT.
    C. P/PRCS.
    D. RCPT.

12. One of the most recent achievements accomplished by the *Respiratory Care* journal is the acceptance in _____, the principle bibliographic database of the National Library of Medicine and its online counterpart, MEDLINE.
    A. *Anesthesiology*
    B. *Index Medicus*
    C. *Chest*
    D. *American Review of Respiratory Disease*

13. The official scientific journal for respiratory therapists is:
    A. *Respiratory Care*.
    B. *Respiratory Therapy*.
    C. *American Review of Respiratory Disease*.
    D. *Chest*.

14. Which of the following is a characteristic of a critical thinker?
    A. Well-informed
    B. Flexible
    C. Inquisitive
    D. All of the above

15. All of the following are functions of the ARCF *except*:
    A. bestow awards.
    B. recognize education and literary contributions.
    C. support scholarly investigations.
    D. provide medical direction.

16. BOMA is an organization:
    A. formed by respiratory therapists.
    B. responsible for the accreditation of respiratory care educational programs.
    C. that provides medical direction and support for respiratory therapists.
    D. that reviews licensure applications from respiratory therapists.

CHAPTER 2

Professional Organizations

1. The American Association for Respiratory Care (AARC) was founded in 1946 and was originally called _____. Funding for the operation of AARC comes from _____, advertising, and revenues from meetings and conventions.
   A. Inhalation Therapy Association; membership dues
   B. American Association for Inhalation Therapy; membership dues
   C. American Association for Respiratory Therapy; federal and state grants
   D. Association for Inhalation Therapy; federal and state grants

2. The AARC consistently provides some of the _____ benefits to its 30,000+ members while keeping the membership dues one of the _____ in the United States.
   A. highest; highest
   B. highest; lowest
   C. lowest, highest
   D. lowest; lowest

3. The governing body of the AARC is its:
   A. president.
   B. executive director.
   C. board of directors.
   D. members.

4. Members of the respiratory care state societies are represented by the:
   A. members of the House of Delegates.
   B. state president.
   C. speaker of the House of Delegates.
   D. general membership.

5. The Board of Medical Advisors elects one representative from each of the following professional medical organizations *except*:
   A. American Society of Anesthesiologists (ASA) and American College of Chest Physicians (ACCP).
   B. American Thoracic Society (ATS) and Society of Critical Care Medicine (SCCM).
   C. American Lung Association (ALA) and American Cancer Society.
   D. A and B.

6. There are _____ specialty sections available to members or others who have an interest in a specialty of respiratory care such as education, home care, transport, and perinatal/pediatric.
   A. six
   B. seven
   C. eight
   D. nine

7. Information on membership, education, employment, and other useful resources and links may be found at the AARC official website:
   A. http://www.aarc.com
   B. http://www.aarc.edu
   C. http://www.aarc.org
   D. http://www.aarc.net

8. The AARC has seven standing committees. In addition to strategic planning, the other standing committees include all of the following *except*:
   A. bylaws and elections.
   B. executive and financial.
   C. judicial and program.
   D. education and management.

9. One of the purposes for appointing chairs of specialty sections having 1000 or more active members to serve as an at-large board of directors is to allow growth of the AARC through:
   A. recruitment of more specialty section members.
   B. potential inclusion of new associations and specialties.
   C. increasing its revenue.
   D. sharing of resources.

10. The National Board for Respiratory Care (NBRC) uses periodic assessment of the actual _____ before developing or revising an exam.
    A. clinical practice of respiratory care
    B. number of respiratory therapists
    C. pass rate on previous exams
    D. cost analysis

11. There are five credentialing exams (two entry level and three advanced) offered by the NBRC. In addition to the perinatal/pediatric respiratory care specialist (PPRCS) credential, the other advanced practice credentials are:
    A. CRT and RRT.
    B. CPFT and RPFT.
    C. CRT and CPFT.
    D. RRT and RPFT.

12. The national accreditation agency for respiratory care educational programs is:
    A. AARC.
    B. CoARC.
    C. NBRC.
    D. ACCP.

13. In addition to annual reports and self-study, each respiratory therapy educational program undergoes a(n) _____ before accreditation or reaccreditation.
    A. phone interview
    B. on-site visit
    C. written evaluation
    D. background check

14. The National Association for Medical Direction of Respiratory Care (NAMDRC):
    A. offers membership to pulmonary medicine physicians only.
    B. offers membership to nonphysicians.
    C. is comprised of medical directors of respiratory care at hospitals.
    D. is comprised of medical directors of respiratory care educational programs.

Questions 15 to 19: Match the professional organizations in Column I with the respective professional journals in Column II. Use each answer ONCE.

Column I

15. American Association for Respiratory Care

16. American College of Chest Physicians (ACCP)

17. Society of Critical Care Medicine (SCCM)

18. American Society of Anesthesiologists (ASA)

19. American Thoracic Society (ATS)

Column II

A. *Anesthesiology*
B. *Critical Care Medicine*
C. *Chest*
D. *American Journal of Respiratory and Critical Care Medicine*
E. *Respiratory Care*

20. Which of the following medical professional organizations accept special membership from nonphysician health care practitioners?
    A. American College of Chest Physicians (ACCP) and Society of Critical Care Medicine (SCCM)
    B. American Society of Anesthesiologists (ASA) and American Thoracic Society (ATS)
    C. American College of Chest Physicians (ACCP) and American Thoracic Society (ATS)
    D. Society of Critical Care Medicine (SCCM) and American Society of Anesthesiologists (ASA)

CHAPTER 3 Health Care Trends and Evolving Roles of Respiratory Care Professionals

1. Cutting costs is one of the major issues of health care reform. Other issues include all of the following *except*:
   A. improving distribution of resources.
   B. improving quality of health care.
   C. evaluating effectiveness of using measurable outcomes.
   D. developing more new medical technologies.

2. _____ payment system is a fee-for-service system and it _____ the health care providers to do more tests and treatments for the patient.
   A. Retrospective; rewards
   B. Retrospective; discourages
   C. Prospective; rewards
   D. Prospective; discourages

3. A student asks you to explain the meaning of *managed care*. You might include in your explanation all of the following terms *except*:
   A. diagnostic-related groups
   B. retrospective payment system
   C. health maintenance organization
   D. preferred provider organization

4. "Graying of America" is a demographic trend showing that health care providers will be working with a greater number of _____ patients in the near future.
   A. sicker
   B. poorer
   C. older
   D. meaner

Questions 5 to 8: Match the factors affecting the health care trend in Column I with the brief descriptions in Column II. Use each answer ONCE.

Column I

5. Epidemiologic factor

6. Demographic factor

7. Sociologic factor

8. Technologic factor

Column II

A. Continuing development in medical procedures, devices, drugs, etc.

B. Increasing complexity in the number and types of patients/illnesses

C. Increasing sensitivity toward the way individuals think, feel, and act about all aspects of life

D. Changing characteristics in the age, ethnicity, economic status, and geographic distribution of the population

9. An ideal educational process is one that trains health care professionals to acquire skills and competencies:
   A. in new technologies.
   B. in new technological advances.
   C. for today.
   D. for the future.

10. _____ is an important issue facing health care reform.
    A. Access to health care
    B. Quality health care at a reasonable cost
    C. Patient satisfaction
    D. All of the above

11. The beginning of respiratory therapy clinical practice can be traced to:
    A. IPPB therapy.
    B. oxygen therapy.
    C. home care.
    D. critical care.

12. Nontraditional roles for respiratory therapy can be described as a(n) _____ work environment _____ the acute care hospital setting.
    A. new; within
    B. new; outside
    C. identical; within
    D. identical; outside

13. The emergence of nontraditional roles for respiratory therapy has been linked to all of the following factors *except*:
    A. inflation.
    B. changes in reimbursement strategies.
    C. aging of the patient population.
    D. cost difference between acute and subacute care.

14. Diagnosis and treatment of sleep-related problems is called:
    A. polygraph.
    B. EEG.
    C. stress testing.
    D. polysomnography.

15. The typical job setting in _____ requires a therapist to work in a diverse environment and with a variety of people.
    A. polysomnography
    B. diagnostic testing
    C. home health care
    D. education

16. A patient asks you to describe the work setting in subacute care. You would tell him that in subacute care, a therapist:
    A. relies on frequent patient assessment and monitoring.
    B. uses a variety of disease prevention techniques.
    C. performs procedures similar to home health care.
    D. performs a variety of diagnostic procedures.

Questions 17 to 19: Match the three phases of a typical pulmonary rehabilitation program in Column I with the respective activities in Column II. Use each answer ONCE.

Column I   Column II

17. Phase I   A. The therapist evaluates the patient and provides follow-up care and long-term maintenance.
18. Phase II
19. Phase III   B. The patient undergoes cardiopulmonary testing, answers questions relating to his or her background, lifestyle, and variety of needs.
              C. The patient receives instruction on topics such as anatomy, disease, medications, equipment, etc.; learns to do prescribed exercises.

20. Mr. Lange, a patient with COPD, asks you to describe a wellness program available to patients with chronic lung diseases. You would explain to him that a wellness program uses different strategies to do all of the following *except*:
    A. maintaining good health.
    B. keeping a healthy diet.
    C. finding the best physician.
    D. exercising and relaxing.

21. Daily clinical review, working with insurance companies, disease prevention, and patient education are some of the duties of a:
    A. case manager.
    B. home care specialist.
    C. respiratory therapist.
    D. polysomnographer.

22. In order to become proficient in researching all aspects of respiratory care, it is essential to have:
    A. appropriate academic credentials.
    B. appropriate professional credentials.
    C. extensive experience and strong clinical background in the area of research.
    D. plenty of free time.

CHAPTER 4 Critical Thinking and Problem-Based Learning in Respiratory Care

1. The ability of an individual to think critically and solve problems has been identified by the _____ to be an essential skill in the respiratory care profession.
   A. American Association for Respiratory Care (AARC)
   B. National Board for Respiratory Care (NBRC)
   C. Committee on Accreditation of Respiratory Care (CoARC)
   D. all of the above

2. A student asks you to explain the meaning of *problem-based learning*. You would explain to him that problem-based learning includes all of the following elements *except*:
   A. problem-solving strategies.
   B. reflection on past experiences.
   C. logical reasoning skills.
   D. recall of factual information.

3. Based on the illustration below, "The Interrelationship of Skills for Critical Thinking in Practice," there are up to _____ components of thinking skills that are required for an individual to link a previous situation to a present situation.
   A. 4
   B. 7
   C. 9
   D. 11

4. As you are getting ready to intubate a patient in the emergency department, the patient suddenly goes into respiratory arrest. This situation calls for _____ skill in order to initiate appropriate steps.
   A. reflecting: "past think"
   B. communicating: "people think"
   C. troubleshooting: "technical think"
   D. prioritizing: "rapid think"

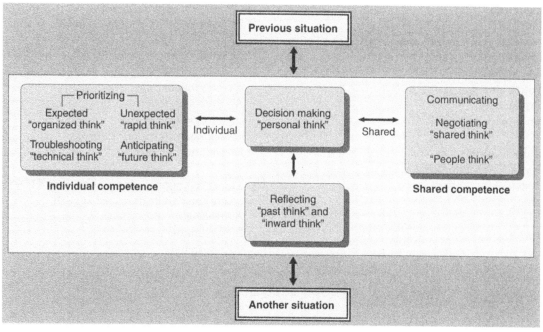

The interrelationship of skills for critical thinking in practice. (From Mishoe SC, Martin S: Critical thinking in the laboratory. *The Learning Series* 1994; 6(4): 1-63.)

5. _____ requires an individual to think ahead and envision potential problems.
   A. Anticipation
   B. Communication
   C. Reflection
   D. Prioritization

6. The ability of a therapist to identify and correct a malfunctioning blood gas analyzer is called:
   A. anticipation.
   B. troubleshooting.
   C. negotiation.
   D. prioritization.

7. While talking with your patient, you find out that he has not been taking his antibiotics as prescribed. In order to share this information with his physician, you need to have mastery of _____ skill.
   A. negotiation
   B. prioritization
   C. communication
   D. reflection

8. Negotiation is the initiation of discussion to _____ others, especially those with an opposing view.
   A. influence
   B. confront
   C. argue with
   D. disagree with

9. The effectiveness of an individual's negotiation skill is greatly influenced by one's ability to:
   A. make decisions.
   B. plan ahead.
   C. troubleshoot.
   D. communicate.

10. Decision-making skill requires careful analysis of all of the following information *except*:
    A. factual information.
    B. conflicting alternatives.
    C. past experiences.
    D. assurance of total success.

11. Which of the following does NOT describe the characteristics of a "critical thinker"?
    A. Well-informed
    B. Cunning
    C. Flexible
    D. Inquisitive

12. Mr. Kingsten is known to have learned from many of his past mistakes. This statement speaks well for his ability to:
    A. plan ahead.
    B. negotiate.
    C. reflect.
    D. troubleshoot.

13. An instructor is learning to integrate critical thinking into one of her RT courses. She should:
    A. develop a set of learning objectives for some of the students.
    B. promote active learning by students.
    C. use daily lesson plans in the classroom.
    D. copy research articles for students.

14. In a traditional classroom, all of the following learning and teaching strategies are highly structured, *except*:
    A. presentation of factual information.
    B. time for questions and discussion.
    C. use of laboratory time.
    D. delivery of lecture content.

15. _____ is an effective teaching and learning model designed to enhance self-learning and critical thinking.
    A. Problem-based learning
    B. Classroom lectures
    C. Laboratory exercises
    D. Clinical practicums

16. Problem-based learning is _____-centered and is suitable for _____ instruction.
    A. student; individualized
    B. student; group or individualized
    C. teacher; individualized
    D. teacher; group or individualized

17. In a typical problem-based course in respiratory care, students are given _____ that gradually unfolds over several group sessions.
    A. a research topic
    B. a lesson plan
    C. textbook and reference sources
    D. a clinical problem

18. The expert person using problem-based learning in a course can best be described as a(n):
    A. teacher.
    B. facilitator.
    C. researcher.
    D. innovator.

19. _____ learning is the key to success in problem-based learning.
    A. Active
    B. Passive
    C. Rote
    D. Guided

20. During problem-based learning sessions, _____ provides each individual a chance to develop the following skills: communication, negotiation, reflection on ideas and actions.
    A. group discussion
    B. reading of problem-based learning script
    C. individual research
    D. recording information for the problem-based learning session

21. Evaluation of students in problem-based learning may include:
    A. peer evaluation.
    B. ability to develop hypotheses and solutions.
    C. types and quality of presentation and discussion.
    D. all of the above.

CHAPTER 5

Ethics of Health Care Delivery

1. *Ethics* is the study of decision-making process a person takes in:
   A. avoiding mistakes.
   B. making medical decisions.
   C. determining possible options.
   D. determining right from wrong.

2. Which of the following statements is believed to be valid concerning a person's value system?
   A. Cultural differences do not affect a person's value system.
   B. Gender differences do not affect a person's value system.
   C. Life experiences may shape or change a person's value system.
   D. A person's value system is inherited at birth.

3. According to common ethical thinking, _____ has (have) the strongest influence on a person's ethical orientation and the decision-making process.
   A. personal principles or values
   B. financial well-being
   C. education
   D. law and order

4. When a person makes a decision not to steal because he believes stealing from others is the wrong thing to do, this decision is based on:
   A. ethical behavior.
   B. legal behavior.
   C. moral behavior.
   D. personal experience.

5. A decision that is based on legal behavior usually allows the person less _____ than a decision made under the ethical behavior.
   A. right
   B. ability
   C. freedom
   D. time

6. *Legal behavior* means abiding by the:
   A. codes of conduct.
   B. law.
   C. community standard.
   D. common belief.

7. Ethical and legal standards of behavior:
   A. change from time to time.
   B. do not change over time.
   C. are inherited at birth.
   D. cannot be learned.

8. A decision is made to forgo one human cloning experiment and use the money to vaccinate thousands of newborns. This action is based on a type of theory known as:
   A. analysis method.
   B. utilitarianism.
   C. beneficence.
   D. nonmaleficence.

9. Teleological theory is based on _____ and deontological theory is related to _____.
   A. right or wrong; intrinsic characters
   B. right or wrong; extrinsic characters
   C. consequences; intrinsic characters
   D. consequences; extrinsic characters

10. There are five steps to guide a person to use the analysis method to make an ethical decision. The third step in this five-step process is to:
    A. test the possible solutions.
    B. identify the problem.
    C. clarify the problem.
    D. develop possible solutions.

Questions 11 to 17: Match the ethical principles in Column I with the respective meanings in Column II. Use each answer ONCE.

Column I   Column II

11. Beneficence   A. Truth
B. Obligation or faithfulness
12. Nonmaleficence   C. Fairness
D. Right to know only
13. Veracity   E. Do good
F. Self-govern
14. Autonomy   G. Avoid harm

15. Confidentiality

16. Justice

17. Role fidelity

18. *Veracity* means _____ and it is a vital element in establishing _____ between the patient and health care providers.
A. informed consent; autonomy
B. advance directive; confidentiality
C. truth; trust
D. self-govern; role fidelity

19. *Patient's Bill of Rights, informed consent, refusal of treatment,* and *advance directives* are four terms that are related to a person's:
A. personal principle.
B. autonomy.
C. veracity.
D. civil rights.

20. The Patient's Bill of Rights describes a person's _____ during the course of medical care.
A. legal rights
B. rights
C. responsibilities
D. rights and responsibilities

21. Under the Patient's Bill of Rights, the patients are:
A. responsible for providing information related to health status.
B. not responsible for providing information about medical history.
C. not responsible for providing information about previous hospitalizations.
D. not given any rights after signing the release forms.

22. Mr. Jones wishes to specify the kind of medical treatments that he wants or does not want. All of the following legal documents would allow him to do this *except*:
A. living wills.
B. medical power of attorney.
C. advance directive.
D. informed consent.

23. Autonomy and paternalism are in conflict because they both deal with the way a(n) _____ is made.
A. decision
B. informed consent
C. living will
D. Bill of Rights

24. The Hippocratic Oath states: "What I may see or hear in the course of treatment ... I will keep to myself holding such things shameful to be spoken aloud." This describes:
A. autonomy.
B. informed consent.
C. confidentiality.
D. Bill of Rights.

25. Technologies such as fax machines and cellular phones are more likely to improve or increase all of the following *except*:
A. quality of medical care.
B. patient confidentiality.
C. access to patient data.
D. communication.

26. Patient's confidentiality may be breached when:
A. the diagnosis is not life-threatening.
B. you know the patient very well.
C. the patient's safety is at risk.
D. the patient's (or another person's) safety is at risk.

27. The question "How should limited health care resources be distributed?" deals with the:
A. principle of justice.
B. Patient's Bill of Rights.
C. principle of veracity.
D. principle of beneficence.

28. The AARC Statement of Ethics and Professional Conduct reads in part that the respiratory care practitioner should "...refuse to conceal illegal, unethical, or incompetent acts of others." This statement reflects the principle of:
A. nonmaleficence.
B. role fidelity.
C. confidentiality.
D. veracity.

29. A health care professional is accepting finder's fees from a home care company for referring patients to that company. This behavior is in conflict with a person's:

    A. role fidelity.
    B. nonmaleficence.
    C. veracity.
    D. confidentiality.

30. Item 6 of the AARC Statement of Ethics and Professional Conduct, "Provide care without discrimination on any basis, with respect for the rights and dignity of all individuals," refers to the principles of:

    A. justice and veracity.
    B. veracity and autonomy.
    C. nonmaleficence and veracity.
    D. autonomy and justice.

CHAPTER 6

Communication Skills

1. Which of the following statements describes communication?
   A. Communication is a simple and static process.
   B. Effective communication can lead to misunderstanding.
   C. Communication is a vital basic life skill.
   D. Effective communication can be learned.

Questions 2 to 6: Match the levels of communication in Column I with the types and characteristics of communication in Column II. Use each answer ONCE.

Column I

Column II

2. Level five   A. Personal ideas and judgments (self-disclosure, guarded and monitored)

3. Level four   B. Fact reporting (neutral topics, no personal information)

4. Level three   C. Peak communication (intimate, reserved for a selected few)

5. Level two   D. Cliché conversation (simple, shallow, superficial)

6. Level one   E. Feelings and emotions (used with trust and mutual respect)

Questions 7 to 11: Match the levels of communication in Column I with the examples of conversation in Column II. Use each answer ONCE.

Column I

Column II

7. Level five   A. "I don't think Mr. Johns should get the treatments because he smokes too much."

8. Level four

9. Level three   B. "You remember the slumber party at Sue's apartment? It was so much fun while we were roommates in college!"

10. Level two   C. "Hi! Morning!"

11. Level one   D. "I worry a lot about my doctor's appointment, Bob. I coughed up blood this morning."

   E. "It looks like it's going to rain today."

12. The content dimension of communication is related to _____, whereas the relationship dimension deals with _____.
    A. words and information; feelings and emotions
    B. books; friendships
    C. documents; marriages
    D. audiovisual materials; relationships

13. Mr. Lee is trying to establish honesty and trust with his patients. The best strategy is to develop the skills that are closely related to the _____ dimensions of communication.
    A. affective and cognitive
    B. content and relationship
    C. relationship and affective
    D. cognitive and content

14. During a meaningful conversation among two or more people, the senders become the receivers and vice versa. This is called _____ communication.
    A. multidimensional
    B. transactional
    C. open
    D. two-way

15. The process of communication can be separated into seven components. Starting with the sender, list the components in proper sequential order.
    A. sender, channel, message, encoding, decoding, receiver, feedback
    B. sender, decoding, encoding, channel, receiver, feedback, message
    C. sender, encoding, decoding, message, channel, feedback, receiver
    D. sender, message, encoding, channel, decoding, receiver, feedback

16. Sending a message via e-mail or posting it on the bulletin board is not an effective way to communicate since the message may not be read by the intended receiver. This is a problem in the _____ of the message.
    A. sending
    B. encoding
    C. decoding
    D. composing

17. Effective communication occurs when the sender and receiver:
    A. share the same meaning of the message.
    B. have a face-to-face conversation.
    C. use nonverbal clues.
    D. communicate with emotions.

Questions 18 to 23: Match the factors affecting communication in Column I with the examples in Column II. Use each answer ONCE.

Column I

Column II

18. Environmental factor

A. The patient experiences severe pain and is worrying about upcoming surgery.

19. Emotional/sensory factor

B. A therapist rolls her eyes while the department head is talking.

20. Verbal expression

C. A therapist is neatly groomed and wearing clean uniform.

21. Nonverbal clues

22. Intrapersonal factor

D. The therapist uses excessive medical jargon and acronyms while explaining a procedure to a patient.

23. Physical appearance and status

E. There is the continuous sound of alarms in the room where a conversation is taking place.

F. The patient is a foreigner and is unfamiliar to the American culture, values, and experience.

24. As you are getting ready to listen to a patient's breath sounds, you should be mindful that you are approaching the patient's:
    A. public space.
    B. social space.
    C. personal space.
    D. intimate space.

25. In regard to using the five senses (taste, touch, smell, hearing, sight) in multiple-sense learning, most people learn by what we _____ and remember by what we _____.
    A. see; say and do
    B. hear; say
    C. smell; do
    D. hear; say and do

26. Expressions made by the _____ are the strongest representation of a person's inner thoughts.
    A. hands
    B. face
    C. body
    D. feet

27. *Intrapersonal factors* can best be described as attributes that are _____ an individual.
    A. inherited by
    B. learned by
    C. within
    D. expressed by

28. All of the following are considered intrapersonal factors affecting communication *except*:
    A. cultural diversity.
    B. mental acuity.
    C. nonverbal clues.
    D. illiteracy.

29. In some cultures, _____ indicates respect but not always agreement.
    A. a handshake
    B. yes
    C. an "OK" sign by thumb and index finger
    D. eye contact

30. The most common barrier to communication is initiated by the:
    A. sender.
    B. physician.
    C. patient.
    D. supervisor.

31. The most important component in establishing believability is to convey:
    A. meaningful contents.
    B. clear and concise sentences.
    C. appropriate appearance and body language.
    D. strong voice and eye contact.

32. You plan on meeting with your department head to discuss some of your concerns. Prior to scheduling the meeting, you would do all of the following *except*:
    A. expect positive feedback
    B. prepare the message.
    C. find a suitable place to meet.
    D. find a proper time to meet.

33. In regard to the skills of a receiver, _____ is an intellectual act that includes understanding and requires active involvement.
    A. hearing
    B. listening
    C. nonverbal clue
    D. facial expression

34. In addition to the content of a message, the receiver should do all of the following *except*:
    A. judge and provide immediate feedback.
    B. listen to the true intent.
    C. assess nonverbal clues.
    D. check emotional filters.

35. Care, empowerment, trust, and empathy are some qualities or characteristics that are important in the development of a:
    A. working relationship.
    B. nurturing relationship.
    C. therapist-patient interaction.
    D. patient care plan.

36. You are interviewing Mr. Hansen before a pulmonary function study. "What is your weight?" would be a(n) _____ question.
    A. open-ended
    B. leading
    C. closed-ended
    D. clarifying

Questions 37 to 40: Match the types of questions in Column I with the examples in Column II. Use each answer ONCE.

Column I   Column II

37. Open-ended   A. "Did you experience wheezing this morning?"
38. Closed-ended   B. "What do you mean by lots of junk when you experience wheezing?"
39. Leading
40. Clarifying   C. "Tell me about your wheezing episodes."
                   D. "You're using MDIs for your wheezing, aren't you?"

41. You should not use compound questions when interviewing a patient because these questions often lead to:
    A. conflicting answers.
    B. incomplete answers.
    C. more questions.
    D. less accurate information.

CHAPTER 7

Decision Making and the Role of the Consultant

1. The evolving role of respiratory therapists to become decision makers and consultants is historically related to the following developments. List them in chronological order from earliest to latest.
   - I. Overutilization of respiratory care
   - II. Fee-for-service system
   - III. Protocol-based respiratory care
   - A. I, II, III
   - B. I, III, II
   - C. II, I, III
   - D. III, I, II

2. A respiratory therapy student asks you to state the common goal for clinical practice guidelines, respiratory care protocols, and critical pathways. You would tell her that they are intended to do all of the following *except*:
   - A. improve efficiency and reduce costs.
   - B. document effectiveness of health care.
   - C. standardize respiratory care practice.
   - D. expand the scope of respiratory care practice.

3. _____ can best be described as practical documents for general application that consist of specific respiratory care procedures to help standardize care and improve quality of care.
   - A. Respiratory care protocols
   - B. Clinical practice guidelines
   - C. Respiratory care plans
   - D. Critical pathways

4. Advantages of clinical practice guidelines (CPGs) include all of the following *except* that they:
   - A. provide independent respiratory care without the need for physician input.
   - B. help to develop a triage system for proper allocation of patient care.
   - C. define and justify clinical practice.
   - D. improve the consistency of care.

5. Development and application of CPGs may be hindered because of lack of _____. This limitation points to the need for more _____.
   - A. clinical evidence; documentation
   - B. clinical evidence; outcomes research
   - C. credentialed respiratory therapists; aggressive recruiting
   - D. credentialed respiratory therapists; pay increases

6. _____ are flexible patient care plans initiated and carried out by credentialed respiratory therapists.
   - A. Respiratory care plans
   - B. Respiratory care protocols
   - C. Clinical practice guidelines
   - D. Critical pathways

7. The most important attribute of respiratory care protocols is to:
   - A. standardize decision making.
   - B. clarify physician orders.
   - C. reduce costs.
   - D. improve morals.

8. Each respiratory care protocol typically includes a title, purpose, and a description of the intended patient population. In addition, each protocol should include all of the following *except*:
   - A. indications and contraindications.
   - B. projected outcomes.
   - C. guidelines for discontinuance.
   - D. description of insurance coverage and limitations.

Questions 9 to 11: Match the types of respiratory care protocols in Column I with the respective examples in Column II. Use each answer ONCE.

Column I

9. Symptom-specific protocol

10. Patient-specific protocol

11. Diagnosis-specific protocol

Column II

A. Premature neonates
B. Respiratory distress syndrome
C. Wheezing

12. Implementation of respiratory care protocols in a hospital may lead to:
A. an unfavorable working environment.
B. poor patient outcomes.
C. lower cost for patient care.
D. low staff morale.

13. Successful implementation of respiratory care protocols in a hospital should be done in a way that the protocols are carried out in a _____ perspective.
A. decision-making
B. task-oriented
C. financial
D. personnel

14. A medical resident asks you to clarify the concept of respiratory care protocols. You would explain to him that these protocols can best be described as:
A. managed care plans.
B. guidelines to terminate therapy.
C. standing orders.
D. institution-specific patient care plans.

15. A *critical pathway* is a sequence of events:
A. leading to the development of a detailed care plan.
B. during a patient's length of stay.
C. leading to laboratory tests and a diagnosis.
D. describing a patient's condition.

16. The ultimate goal for implementing critical pathways is to:
A. justify more respiratory therapists.
B. expand the scope of practice.
C. improve efficiency.
D. document a patient's living will.

17. All of the following describe the characteristics of critical pathways *except* that they:
A. may be purchased from an outside source.
B. should be developed by those who use them.

C. are developed by an outside source and may be implemented by any hospital.
D. optimize the sequence and timing of patient intervention by health care providers.

18. Critical pathways play an important role in all of the following *except*:
A. clinical practice guidelines.
B. continuous quality improvement (CQI) plans.
C. identification of potential and actual variations in patient response.
D. case management.

19. One common pitfall in the implementation of critical pathways is that:
A. too many health care professionals are involved in the process.
B. too much time is spent in the process of review, preparation, and communication.
C. they require support and commitment from administrators, physicians, and managers.
D. they are adopted without adequate review, preparation, and communication.

Questions 20 to 22: Match the types of outcomes in Column I with the respective examples in Column II. Use each answer ONCE.

Column I

20. Patient outcomes

21. Institutional outcomes

22. Care provider outcomes

Column II

A. Improvement in efficiency and quality of care
B. Reduction in staff member turnover rate
C. Improvement in quality of life

23. In outcomes evaluation, the term _____ is used when a patient does not progress as expected or when an expected outcome does not happen.
A. morbidity
B. variance
C. deviation
D. critical pathway

24. A new employee in respiratory care asks you to explain why the department is keeping track of variance. You would list all of the following reasons *except* that variance may be used to:
A. guide decisions and make changes.
B. minimize overuse of resources.
C. prevent underuse of appropriate resources.
D. determine the real cost for a given diagnosis.

25. *Benchmarking* is a term used to describe the:
    A. average use of resources per diagnosis.
    B. productivity level of staff members.
    C. average length of stay.
    D. most appropriate use of resources per diagnosis.

26. A hospital is developing a plan to deliver certain clinical procedures based on scientific evidence and outcomes data. This is called:
    A. evidence-based medicine.
    B. respiratory care protocols.
    C. critical pathways.
    D. continuous quality improvement.

27. The primary goal of evidence-based medicine is to:
    A. expand the scope of practice.
    B. reduce the number of staff.
    C. implement standing orders.
    D. improve effectiveness of health care.

28. The roles of an internal consultant should include all of the following *except* to:
    A. identify problems.
    B. develop solutions to problems.
    C. implement critical pathways.
    D. communicate results to others.

CHAPTER **8**

Patient Education

1. The Joint Commission on Accreditation of Healthcare Organizations (JCAHO) is a(n) _____ agency and it requires health care organizations to provide _____ to patients as a condition for accreditation.
   A. educational; education
   B. educational; health screening
   C. regulatory; education
   D. regulatory; health screening

2. With the "Graying of America," the number of caregivers _____ medical training has _____ in homes across the United States.
   A. with; increased
   B. with; decreased
   C. without; increased
   D. without; decreased

3. When a patient education program is presented to staff respiratory therapists, the process is called:
   A. patient education.
   B. consumer education.
   C. continuing education.
   D. client education.

4. In _____ education, the learner is almost completely dependent on the health care professional to provide the information that he or she is lacking.
   A. client
   B. patient
   C. consumer
   D. continuing

5. In promoting wellness, an educational program should include all of the following components *except*:
   A. modifying a person's behavior.
   B. motivating a person to practice a healthy lifestyle.
   C. teaching essential information on wellness.
   D. testing for any hidden lung diseases.

6. An ineffective and unsuccessful patient education program is one that relies heavily on the strategy of:
   A. telling the patient about the diagnosis and treatment options.
   B. helping the patient to learn about the disease state.
   C. causing a change in the patient's behavior.
   D. showing the patient how to do things.

7. In regard to patient education, the goals or expectations of the patient and caregiver include all of the following *except*:
   A. obtaining accurate information about the disease.
   B. reducing anxiety and increasing satisfaction with health-related matters
   C. meeting accreditation requirements.
   D. developing ability to make decisions.

8. In patient education, *APIE* means:
   A. atypical pulmonary interstitial emphysema.
   B. a program for independent learning.
   C. a partner in education.
   D. assessment, planning, implementing, evaluation.

9. During a patient training program, you ask the patient to demonstrate the use of a metered dose inhaler. This is called _____ in the process of patient education.
   A. evaluation
   B. assessment
   C. implementation
   D. planning

10. The most common mistake that educators make in a patient training program is failure to _____ the patient's _____.
    A. assess; needs
    B. assess; desires
    C. evaluate; outcome
    D. evaluate; medical condition

11. Locus of control is related to the _____ level of a patient and this is an important element in the process of _____.
    A. educational; learning
    B. motivation; learning
    C. mental; thinking
    D. intellectual; thinking

12. In developing the goals for a patient education program, it is essential that each goal:
    A. meets the need of the patient.
    B. follows the preestablished health model.
    C. uses the PRECEDE-PROCEED model.
    D. incorporates the external locus of control method.

13. "I will help Mr. Jones, a 50-pack-per-year smoker, to lose 100 lbs." is an example that best describes an objective that is:
    A. attainable.
    B. relevant.
    C. having timeline.
    D. measurable.

Questions 14 to 16: Match the types of learning domains in Column I with the anticipated outcomes in Column II. Use each answer ONCE.

Column I

14. Affective

15. Cognitive

16. Psychomotor

Column II

A. The patient is able to explain the process of emphysema and describe the treatment plan.
B. The patient is able to use the metered dose inhaler correctly and as prescribed.
C. The patient is free to share some of his feelings in regard to his terminal illness.

17. The physician asks you to provide instructions to a patient on the use of a metered dose inhaler prior to discharge from the hospital. You would select and use the _____ method in order to engage the patient in active learning.
    A. case study
    B. lecture
    C. drills
    D. demonstration and return demonstration

18. _____ should be used to teach a patient who is being discharged from the hospital in an hour or so.
    A. Lecture
    B. Fact sheet or simple demonstration
    C. Audiovisual presentation
    D. Journal articles

19. A staff respiratory therapist asks you about how to determine if the patient has learned the material specifically tailored to the patient's needs. You would advise him to compare the learning outcomes with the learning _____.
    A. models.
    B. methods.
    C. objectives.
    D. lessons.

20. Evaluation, the last phase in patient education, should be done to encompass the _____ teaching process.
    A. self-learning
    B. entire
    C. end of the
    D. beginning of the

CHAPTER 9

Documentation and Medical Information Management

1. The forms committee in a health care system is responsible for all issues relating to:
   A. patient information.
   B. employee health records.
   C. health care insurance information.
   D. health care regulatory compliance data.

2. Dr. Hines tells a senior respiratory therapy student to add "albuterol MDI 2 puffs Q 4 hr prn" to a patient's daily respiratory care plan. The student should first:
   A. record the verbal order in the patient's chart.
   B. instruct the patient on the proper use of MDI.
   C. ask a staff respiratory therapist to record the verbal order.
   D. ask a staff respiratory therapist to call physician and verify the verbal order.

3. In addition to the patient's name and identification number, a typical verbal order should include all of the following written documentation *except*:
   A. date and time.
   B. patient's consent.
   C. name of physician.
   D. name and credential of person writing the verbal order.

4. A respiratory therapy student asks you the proper method to authenticate verbal orders in a patient's medical record. You would tell her that based one JCAHO requirement, all of the following must be included *except*:
   A. physician signatures on all verbal orders.
   B. names of physicians who gave the verbal orders.
   C. names of persons who carried out the verbal orders.
   D. names of persons who recorded the verbal orders.

5. In regard to a patient's confidentiality, all of following statements are true *except*:
   A. breaching of such information may cause the responsible person to be fired.
   B. breaching of such information may cause the responsible person to face legal action.
   C. the health care provider must consider the patient's need when disclosing patient's medical information.
   D. health care providers may discuss a patient's medical information in the elevator when the door is closed.

6. Due to technological advances, there are many ways that a patient's confidentiality can be put at risk. These technologies include:
   A. e-mail, voice mail, phone, and pager.
   B. facsimile (fax) machine and copier.
   C. computer display and printer.
   D. all of the above.

7. Authorization to release medical information is not permitted when it is made by the:
   A. patient.
   B. patient's power of attorney.
   C. patient's physician.
   D. executor of the patient's estate.

8. A complete medical record may consist of:
   A. paper hardcopy to include physician order, laboratory results, and progress notes.
   B. monitoring strips and audio recordings.
   C. photographs and videotapes.
   D. all of the above.

9. Once fully developed, the computer-based patient record (CPR) system will be able to:
   A. offer easy access to clinical data.
   B. eliminate paper hardcopies of medical records.
   C. provide diagnosis and treatment options.
   D. reduce breaching of patient confidentiality.

10. Electronic signature is essentially a unique _____ that identifies the _____ of an electronic medium.
    A. code or password; location
    B. code or password; user
    C. symbol; location
    D. symbol; user

Questions 11 to 13: Match the types of information security controls in Column I with the selected functions in Column II. Use each answer ONCE.

Column I   Column II

11. Management control   A. Identification and authentication
12. Operational control B. User awareness and training
13. Technical control   C. Security policies

14. The report released by the National Research Council in 1997 provides guidelines on protecting:
    A. patient confidentiality.
    B. electronic health care information.
    C. health care workers from infectious diseases.
    D. federal and state employees from malpractice lawsuits.

15. Sending a patient's medical information via facsimile (fax) may be done:
    A. to save postage.
    B. regardless patient's medical history.
    C. to provide immediate patient care.
    D. only with a patient's consent.

16. Medicare requires that patient medical records and other medical documents and images be kept for a minimum of _____ years.
    A. 1
    B. 5
    C. 10
    D. 30

17. The Occupational Safety and Health Administration (OSHA) requires that employee medical records be kept for the period of employment plus _____ years.
    A. 1
    B. 5
    C. 10
    D. 30

18. Medical records should not be destroyed if they involve:
    A. investigation, audit, or litigation.
    B. Medicare or Medicaid claims.
    C. high-risk patients.
    D. written incident reports.

19. As you are treating Ms. Jones, her roommate gets out of bed and accidentally falls. You should fill out a(n):
    A. accident report form.
    B. incident report form.
    C. lawsuit on behalf of the roommate.
    D. medical and liability waiver on behalf of Ms. Jones.

CHAPTER 10

Assessing Outcomes

1. You are assisting the RT department to implement outcomes assessment. It is important to educate others in the department that the goals and benefits of outcomes assessment include all of the following *except* to:
   A. prevent adverse effects of patient care.
   B. improve professional image.
   C. improve clinical quality and patient service.
   D. enhance cost effectiveness and appropriateness of care.

Questions 2 to 5: Match the examples of clinical outcomes in Column I with the types of outcomes in Column II. You may use any answer MORE THAN ONCE.

Column I	Column II
2. SpO$_2$ change during titration of F$_I$O$_2$	A. Short-term outcome
	B. Long-term outcome

3. Number of patients using oxygen at home 10 weeks after discharge from hospital

4. Mortality rate of patient one year following discontinuance of mechanical ventilation

5. Changes in heart rate during SVN therapy with a bronchodilator

6. Outcomes research is not done to improve:
   A. patient care.
   B. patient outcomes.
   C. cost effectiveness.
   D. department prestige.

7. Individuals or groups that influence outcomes assessment in health care include:
   A. insurers, government, business, and industry.
   B. regulatory and provider organizations.
   C. practitioners and consumers.
   D. all of the above.

8. Surveys, tests, and questionnaires are some useful tools for:
   A. outcomes assessment.
   B. patient care.
   C. hospital accreditation.
   D. insurance reimbursement.

9. _____ is the accreditation agency that assesses and determines which hospitals, home health care companies, and nursing homes may get reimbursement for taking care of Medicare patients.
   A. Joint Commission on Accreditation of Hospitals (JCAH)
   B. Joint Commission on Accreditation of Healthcare Organizations (JCAHO)
   C. Health Maintenance Organization (HMO)
   D. Health Care Finance Agency (HCFA)

10. Outcomes may be classified or categorized by:
   A. time lines (immediate, short-term, long-term).
   B. service, quality, and cost.
   C. continuum of care and perspective.
   D. all of the above.

Questions 11 to 14: Match the types of study in Column I with the types of outcomes in Column II. You may use any answer MORE THAN ONCE.

Column I

11. Patient satisfaction

12. Rate of patient readmission

13. Number of patients who died

14. Opinion of visitors

Column II

A. Quantitative outcome
B. Qualitative outcome

15. *Continuum of care* refers to a category of conditions that is related to:
    A. home care plan.
    B. pulmonary rehabilitation program.
    C. adverse patient outcomes.
    D. universal insurance coverage.

Questions 16 to 19: Match the outcomes classified by perspective in Column I with the examples in Column II. Use each answer ONCE.

Column I

16. Clinical perspective

17. Functional perspective

18. Financial perspective

19. Perceptual perspective

Column II

A. Efficient use of resources
B. Patient satisfaction with outcomes
C. Improvement of physical performance
D. Response to respiratory care treatment

20. Refer to the asthma study in the textbook that involves two school districts. The outcomes of asthma education may be assessed by evaluating the changes that have occurred in:
    A. the school district that received the asthma education program.
    B. the school district that did not receive the asthma education program.
    C. all other school districts in the state that received the asthma education program.
    D. A and B.

21. In the "Disease Prevention" section of the textbook chapter, the smoking cessation program showed positive outcomes because it:
    A. reduced the number of smokers.
    B. reduced the future medical expenditures.
    C. reduced the number of smoking-related illnesses.
    D. all of the above.

CHAPTER 11

Health Care Reimbursement

Questions 1 to 4: Match the major functions of health care system in the United States in Column I with the related organizations or individuals in Column II. Use each answer ONCE.

Column I

1. Financing of health care

2. Insurance for health care coverage

3. Delivery of health care

4. Payment for health care provided

Column II

A. Government, managed care organizations, patients

B. Physicians, therapists, nurses, etc.

C. Government, employers

D. Insurance companies or managed care organizations

Questions 5 to 8: Match the major functions of health care system in the United States in Column I with the roles in Column II. Use each answer ONCE.

Column I

5. Financing of health care

6. Insurance for health care coverage

7. Delivery of health care

8. Payment for health care provided

Column II

A. Reimbursement and disbursement of funds

B. Purchase of health insurance

C. Protection against risk

D. Provision of services

9. Who is considered the third-party payer among the following stakeholders in health care reimbursement?
   A. Patient
   B. Insurer
   C. Taxpayer
   D. Provider

10. Downsizing, decentralizing, restructuring, and reengineering are processes that directly affect the _____ and they are intended to _____.
    A. patients; reduce cost
    B. patients; improve quality of health care
    C. providers; reduce cost
    D. providers; improve quality of health care

11. To minimize financial harm to the health care industry, considerable pressure has been applied to the _____ to increase productivity, improve patient satisfaction, and reduce cost.
    A. federal and state agencies
    B. patients
    C. insurers
    D. providers

12. Reduction in health insurance premiums, copayments, or deductibles in exchange for smoking cessation and other healthy lifestyle behaviors is targeted toward the _____ for the purpose of reducing the financial burden on the health care system.
    A. providers
    B. patients
    C. insurers
    D. federal and state agencies·

13. Which of the following factors is *least* likely responsible for the rising health care costs in the 1990s?
    A. Technological advances
    B. Epidemics and deadlier diseases
    C. Population growth
    D. General and medical price inflation

Questions 14 to 16: Match the terms related to rising health care costs in Column I with the descriptions in Column II. Use ONLY THREE answers.

Column I   Column II

14. Fragmentation

15. Defense medicine

16. Fraud

A. Overuse of medical resources in response to fear of litigation and malpractice lawsuits
B. Inadequate medical insurance
C. Duplication of unnecessary services due to lack of coordination among providers
D. Health care provided to inmates
E. Improper and illegal claims made for the purpose of financial or personal gain

17. _____ payment system is one that reimburses the providers for the total costs of covered benefits provided to the patient. It is _____ today to most Americans.
   A. Prospective; widely available
   B. Retrospective; widely available
   C. Prospective; no longer available
   D. Retrospective; no longer available

18. Shared risk and shared losses are the working concept behind the development of:
   A. health insurance.
   B. Medicare Part A.
   C. Medicare Part B.
   D. Medicaid.

19. In regard to the health care reimbursement programs provided by the U.S. government,
   A. Medicare and Medicaid were enacted in 1935.
   B. Medicare Part A is for hospital coverage.
   C. Medicare Part B is for skilled nursing facility coverage.
   D. Medicaid provides coverage for elderly.

20. Prospective payment system (PPS) sets a _____ payment for the _____ for admission to the hospital.
   A. fixed; primary reason
   B. fixed; primary reason and secondary complications
   C. variable; primary reason
   D. variable; primary reason and secondary complications

Questions 21 to 23: Match the acronyms in Column I with the meanings related to health care reimbursement in Column II. Use ONLY THREE answers.

Column I   Column II

21. CPT code

22. RBRVS

23. PMPM

A. The monthly fee paid by each enrollee
B. RT procedure for pulmonary hygiene
C. A government, employers
D. Physician reimbursement under the PPS
E. A number assigned to each medical procedure

24. *Capitation* is a term that describes a _____ amount of money paid to providers _____.
   A. variable; regardless of the services provided
   B. variable; for the services provided
   C. fixed; regardless of the services provided
   D. fixed; for the services provided

25. The general characteristics of a health maintenance organization (HMO) include all of the following *except*:
   A. health services are provided by participating providers.
   B. providers get a fixed fee for services provided.
   C. preventive services are emphasized.
   D. quality of services is left up to the providers.

26. In general, the _____ model of HMO offers the greatest number of participating physicians and health care providers.
   A. staff
   B. group
   C. network
   D. independent practice association

27. Preferred provider organizations (PPOs) differ from HMOs in that PPOs offer enrollees:
   A. a discount.
   B. more choices of participating providers.
   C. selection and use of nonparticipating providers.
   D. all of the above.

28. _____ allow a person to choose and use a nonparticipating provider at the time of need.
   A. PPOs
   B. Point-of-service plans (POSs)
   C. HMOs
   D. Exclusive provider organizations

29. The health care plan offered by exclusive provider organizations (EPOs) differs from HMOs, PPOs, and POSs in that the enrollees must use the _____ allowed in the plan and _____.
    A. hospitals; limited choices of physician are available
    B. physicians; limited choices of hospitals are available
    C. hospitals; no choices are allowed
    D. hospitals; and physicians, no choices are allowed

30. The major drawback of "fee for service" and "cost plus" reimbursements is that providers are:
    A. rewarded for providing more services.
    B. overworked due to increased patient load.
    C. paid a fixed rate and the quality of care is lowered as a result.
    D. penalized for cutting costs.

31. In prospective reimbursement, the fees that the providers receive are:
    A. fixed at a predetermined amount before services are rendered.
    B. based on the types and number of services rendered.
    C. variable based on the length of stay.
    D. not determined until the patient's discharge.

32. Diagnostic-related group (DRG) system is a reimbursement method based on _____ for a particular _____ established at the time of admission.
    A. individual services; diagnosis
    B. individual services; length of stay
    C. bundled services; diagnosis
    D. bundled services; length of stay

33. Under the diagnostic-related group (DRG) system, a hospital's revenue is typically _____ when the patient is treated and discharged _____ than average.
    A. increased; later
    B. increased; earlier
    C. unchanged, later
    D. unchanged, earlier

34. Which of the following respiratory care services is most likely to carry bundled charges?
    A. Arterial blood gases
    B. Pulmonary rehabilitation
    C. Daily mechanical ventilation
    D. Endotracheal intubation

35. Copayment is the _____ for health benefits received and it is paid directly by the _____.
    A. entire fee; insurance company
    B. partial fee; patient
    C. entire; government
    D. partial fee; insurance company

36. In the near future, the health care system in the United States will likely see:
    A. employer-based insurance to remain the dominant source of health insurance.
    B. wellness and preventive medicine to become more popular.
    C. more patients to receive their health care at home.
    D. all of the above.

CHAPTER 12

Evaluating and Accessing Medical Information

1. Textbooks:
   A. contain the most current information.
   B. are updated with new editions every two years.
   C. serve as the primary source of information in an educational program.
   D. undergo an extensive peer-review process.

2. Journals:
   A. contain information that is similar to textbooks.
   B. are updated with new editions every two years.
   C. serve as the primary source of information in an educational program.
   D. undergo an extensive peer-review process.

3. In addition to *Respiratory Care*, all of the following journals are related to the respiratory care profession *except*:
   A. *Chest*.
   B. *American Journal of Respiratory and Critical Care Medicine*.
   C. *Critical Care Medicine*.
   D. *Respiratory Update*.

4. Which of the following statements is true in regard to journals?
   A. There are about 10,000 scholarly journals.
   B. The quality of journal articles is related to the number of subscriptions.
   C. The most well-known person is listed as the first author in a journal article.
   D. Journals contain the most current published information.

Questions 5 to 9: Match the types of studies in Column I with the descriptions in Column II. Use each answer ONCE.

Column I

5. Case report
6. Case control
7. Cohort
8. Clinical trials
9. Surveys

Column II

A. A comparison of patients (affected versus control) from a number of cases
B. A study to gather opinions or behaviors
C. A study designed to test a new treatment or therapy
D. A detailed report based on observations
E. A long-term study that involves follow-up with a large number of patients

10. IMRAD stands for the:
    A. components of a medical report.
    B. type of medical research.
    C. type of clinical trial.
    D. name of a respiratory care journal.

11. Which of the following statements is accurate in regard to abstracts?
    A. An abstract serves as a brief description of the study.
    B. An abstract allows the reader to draw conclusions quickly.
    C. Conference abstracts undergo extensive peer-review.
    D. An abstract contains enough details for a critical analysis of the study.

12. The _____ section of a journal article provides information to others so they can verify, repeat, or expand on the study.
    A. introduction
    B. methods
    C. results
    D. conclusions

13. The control group of an experiment:
    A. serves as a dependent variable.
    B. has fewer subjects than the study group.
    C. receives the new treatment.
    D. does not receive the new treatment.

14. Randomization is a process in the research study to eliminate:
    A. blinding effect.
    B. crossovers.
    C. bias.
    D. variables.

15. When the researchers and study subjects are not aware which treatments are being used, the study is called:
    A. single blind.
    B. single crossover.
    C. double blind.
    D. double crossover.

16. If a researcher wants to test the effects of a new drug on subjects of the same age, gender, and disease state, a _____ design should be considered.
    A. retrospective
    B. double blind
    C. crossover
    D. matching

17. Entrance and exclusion criteria of a research study:
    A. must be stipulated before the study.
    B. are not reported in a clinical trial article.
    C. may be modified during the study.
    D. all of the above.

18. Prospective studies:
    A. look at records and study what has been done.
    B. reduce the likelihood of bias.
    C. require a clear proposal and research plan.
    D. all of the above.

19. The primary function of an institutional review board is to protect the _____ of the research study:
    A. researchers.
    B. participants.
    C. institution.
    D. department managers.

20. A statistically significant result means that the results can be applied to:
    A. the study itself.
    B. other settings with the same participants.
    C. other settings under similar conditions.
    D. other studies with different designs.

21. *Median* is defined as the _____ value when the measurements are listed in sequential order. For example, the median is _____ for the following set of numbers: 11, 12, 12, 12, 13, 13, 14, 15, 16.
    A. average; 13
    B. middle; 13
    C. most frequent; 12
    D. highest; 16

22. *Mode* is defined as the _____ value. The mode is _____ for the following numbers: 11, 12, 12, 12, 13, 13, 14, 15, 16.
    A. average; 13
    B. lowest; 11
    C. middle; 13
    D. most frequent; 12

23. *Mean* is defined as the _____ value. The mean is _____ for the following numbers: 11, 12, 12, 12, 13, 13, 14, 15, 16.
    A. most frequent; 12
    B. highest; 16
    C. average; 13
    D. middle; 13

24. Null hypothesis is based on the assumption that the treatment:
    A. has a significant effect on the participants in the control group.
    B. has a significant effect on the participants in the testing group.
    C. does not have a significant effect on the participants in the control group.
    D. does not have a significant effect on the participants in the testing group.

25. In research statistics, differences are commonly measured by the _____ and associations are measured using the _____ analysis.
    A. normal distribution curve; correlation
    B. t-test; correlation
    C. skewed distribution curve; normal distribution curve
    D. regression; t-test

26. In regard to statistics, which of the following statements is correct?
    A. Statistical results do not contain errors.
    B. Importance of a study should be based on statistics alone.
    C. Clinical value of the findings should be evaluated along with the statistics.
    D. Researchers are also be experts in statistics.

27. References in a research paper are listed to:
    A. establish credibility of the study.
    B. satisfy the peer-review process.
    C. get published.
    D. provide readers sources for further information.

28. In the sample citation below, the volume number is _____. Doe, J. J. Strategies to improve reading skills. *Learning Daily* 2002;111(11): 1–10.
    A. 2002
    B. 111
    C. 11
    D. 1–10

29. Which of the following is not a searchable database for medical information available via the Internet?
    A. MEDLINE
    B. PubMed
    C. Grateful Med
    D. IMRAD

30. To obtain useful and current information on evidence-based medicine, one should use:
    A. CINAHL.
    B. MEDLINE.
    C. the Cochrane Library.
    D. MD Consult.

CHAPTER 13

Mathematical Aspects of Respiratory Care

Questions 1 to 8: *Match the types of measurements in Column I with the proper units of measurement in Column II. You may use any answer MORE THAN ONCE.*

Column I

1. Pressure limits

2. F_IO_2

3. Compliance

4. Electrolytes (e.g., HCO_3^-)

5. Ratios (e.g., FEV_1/FVC, V_D/V_T)

6. PaO_2

7. pH

8. Oxygen flow via nasal cannula

Column II

A. no units
B. mL/cmH$_2$O
C. mm Hg
D. mEq/L
E. cmH$_2$O
F. L/min

9. Three consecutive peak flow measurements are obtained: 260 L/min, 270 L/min, 280 L/min. You would report _____ as the peak flow value since these measurements likely have indeterminate errors.
A. 260 L/min
B. 270 L/min
C. 280 L/min
D. 810 L/min

Questions 10 to 13: *Match the types of metric measurements in Column I with the standard base units of measurement in Column II. Use ONLY FOUR answers.*

Column I

10. Length

11. Weight

12. Volume

13. Temperature

Column II

A. Degrees Celsius
B. Pounds
C. Inch
D. Gram
E. Liter
F. Gallon
G. Meter

Questions 14 to 17: *Match the metric prefixes in Column I with the mathematical notations in Column II. Use ONLY FOUR answers.*

Column I

14. Centi-

15. Deci-

16. Kilo-

17. Milli-

Column II

A. 10^3
B. 10^2
C. 10^1
D. 10^{-1}
E. 10^{-2}
F. 10^{-3}
G. 10^{-4}

18. In arterial blood gases, PCO_2 (partial pressure of carbon dioxide) carries a unit of _____ and a measurement of 32.4 may be rounded to _____.
A. cmH$_2$O; 32
B. cmH$_2$O; 33
C. mm Hg; 32
D. mm Hg; 33

19. As you are reviewing a patient's laboratory reports, you notice that the most recent WBC (white blood counts) shows 1.4×10^3. You may infer that the patient's WBC is:
    A. 140 cells/cm^3.
    B. 1,400 cells/cm^3.
    C. 14,000 cells/cm^3.
    D. 140,000 cells/cm^3.

20. Δ is a mathematical symbol meaning:
    A. add to.
    B. subtract from.
    C. change in.
    D. delete from.

21. The mathematical expression for logarithms is based on powers of _____. Thus, the log for 100 (or 10^2) is _____.
    A. 10, 2
    B. 10, 10
    C. 100, 2
    D. 100, 10

22. Based on the precedence of mathematical operations, which portion of the Henderson-Hasselbach (pH) equation below should be done first?

    $$pH = 6.1 + \log[HCO_3^-/(PaCO_2 \times 0.03)]$$

    A. $\log HCO_3^-$
    B. $6.1 + \log$
    C. $HCO_3^-/PaCO_2$
    D. $PaCO_2 \times 0.03$

23. During controlled mechanical ventilation, a patient has an inspiratory (I) time of 1 second and an inspiratory:expiratory (I:E) ratio of 1:2. The expiratory (E) time is therefore _____ and the respiratory rate (RR) is _____.
    A. 1 sec.; 30/min
    B. 2 sec.; 20/min
    C. 3 sec.; 15/min
    D. Insufficient data to determine E time and RR

24. What is the area of a square if each side measures 1 inch?
    A. 1 sq. in.
    B. 2 sq. in.
    C. 4 sq. in.
    D. Insufficient data to calculate area of a square

Questions 25 to 28: Match the areas and volumes in Column I with the formulas in Column II. Use ONLY FOUR answers.

Column I

25. Area of a circle

26. Area of a rectangle

27. Volume of a cylinder

28. Volume of a cube

Column II

A. length x height
B. length x height x width
C. pi x radius^2
D. length x pi x radius^2
E. length^2
F. length^3

29. The oxyhemoglobin curve is an example of a _____ curve where its top portion is rather _____ reflecting small changes in the oxygen saturation level over a wide range of PO_2.
    A. parabolic; flat
    B. parabolic; steep
    C. sigmoid; steep
    D. sigmoid; flat

30. In the equation below, P_2 is called a(n):

    $$P_2 = (P_1V_1)/V_2$$

    A. dependent variable
    B. independent variable
    C. function
    D. constant

31. If C (compliance) is constant in the equation $P = V/C$ (where P = pressure and V = volume), which of the following is true?
    A. Pressure and volume would also be constant.
    B. Higher pressure would lead to smaller volume.
    C. Higher pressure would lead to larger volume.
    D. Insufficient information to determine answer.

32. If P (pressure) is constant in the equation $Q = P/R$ (where Q = flow and R = resistance), which of the following is true?
    A. Flow and resistance would also be constant.
    B. Higher resistance would lead to lower flow.
    C. Higher resistance would lead to higher flow.
    D. Insufficient information to determine answer.

33. Differential equations are useful to predict the behavior of the system over a:
    A. surface area.
    B. liquid medium.
    C. gaseous medium.
    D. course of time.

34. In pressure-controlled ventilation, the pressure provided by the ventilator and applied to the patient is used to overcome the:
    A. elastic recoil of the lungs and chest wall.
    B. resistive pressure of the airways.
    C. elastic and resistive pressure of the ventilator circuit.
    D. all of the above.

CHAPTER 14

Application of Physical Principles

1. Which of the following molecules is composed of the same element?
   A. O_2
   B. CO_2
   C. NaCl
   D. H_2O

2. There are _____ states of matter and _____ is the most stable form.
   A. 2; solid
   B. 2; gas
   C. 3; solid
   D. 3; liquid

3. A unit under the SI system, kPa (kilo Pascal), is to measure _____ . In the United States, cm H_2O and mm Hg remain in common use to make similar measurements.
   A. volume
   B. weight
   C. pressure
   D. length

Questions 4 to 8: Match the primary symbols in Column I with the meanings in Column II. Use ONLY FIVE answers.

Column I

Column II

4. P

A. Fraction

B. Compliance

5. F

C. Conductance

D. Pressure

6. V

E. Ratio

F. Resistance

7. C

G. Force

H. Volume

8. R

9. A patient's arterial blood gases show a PO_2 of 100 torr. This is same as:
   A. 100 kPa.
   B. 100 mm Hg.
   C. 100 cm H_2O.
   D. all of the above.

10. A respiratory therapist reports that the patient's compliance has been getting higher over the past few days. This means that the patient's elastance is _____ than before and a _____ pressure is needed to deliver the same volume.
    A. higher; lower
    B. higher; higher
    C. lower; lower
    D. lower; higher

11. A neonate has developed respiratory distress syndrome due to surfactant deficiency. This means that the surface tension in the lungs is _____ than normal and the work of breathing is likely to _____.
    A. higher; increase
    B. higher; decrease
    C. lower; increase
    D. lower; decrease

12. Which of the following temperature readings refer to normal body temperature?
    A. 0° Kelvin; 25° Celsius; 98.6° Fahrenheit
    B. 100° Kelvin; 25° Celsius; 100° Fahrenheit
    C. 273° Kelvin; 37° Celsius; 100° Fahrenheit
    D. 310° Kelvin; 37° Celsius; 98.6° Fahrenheit

13. In pulmonary function testing, the lung volumes recorded at room temperature are converted to volumes at body temperature. This volume-temperature relationship is related to:
    A. Boyle's law.
    B. Charles' law.
    C. Combined gas law.
    D. Gay-Lussac's law.

14. Based on the combined gas law $(P_1 \times V_1)/T_1 = (P_2 \times V_2)/T_2$:
    A. pressure and volume are directly proportional.
    B. pressure and temperature are directly proportional.
    C. volume and temperature are inversely proportional.
    D. all of the above.

15. A patient is using a 40% air-entrainment oxygen mask. At a barometric pressure of 760 mm Hg, the pressure of inspired oxygen, is:
    A. 40 mm Hg.
    B. 304 mm Hg.
    C. 720 mm Hg.
    D. 800 mm Hg.

16. Among other gases, dry air contains about 21% _____ and 0.03% _____.
    A. nitrogen; argon
    B. nitrogen; helium
    C. oxygen; carbon dioxide
    D. oxygen; carbon monoxide

17. At body temperature and 100% saturation, the water vapor pressure is about:
    A. 22 mm Hg.
    B. 29 mm Hg.
    C. 44 mm Hg.
    D. 47 mm Hg.

18. The pressure gauge for compressed _____ in a cylinder does not show the remaining gas content because at the compressed state, these gases are partly in _____ form and do not exert pressure.
    A. carbon monoxide or nitrogen; solid
    B. carbon monoxide or nitrous oxide; liquid
    C. carbon dioxide or nitrogen; solid
    D. carbon dioxide or nitrous oxide; liquid

19. The gram molecular weight for four gases are as follows: helium = 4; carbon dioxide = 44; oxygen = 32; nitrogen = 28. Based on Graham's law alone (not accounting for the diffusion coefficient), _____ has the highest rate of diffusion.
    A. helium
    B. carbon dioxide
    C. oxygen
    D. nitrogen

20. When a gas volume is measured at 37° Celsius, one atmospheric pressure, and 100% humidity, this condition can be described as:
    A. STPD.
    B. ATPD.
    C. ATPS.
    D. BTPS.

21. In spite of being a heavier gas, carbon dioxide diffuses in blood _____ than oxygen because carbon dioxide has a _____ diffusion coefficient.
    A. 19 times faster; higher
    B. 19 times slower; lower
    C. 210 times faster; higher
    D. 210 times slower; lower

22. Based on the Bernoulli Principle, the velocity of a fluid:
    A. increases as it moves through a constriction.
    B. is inversely related to the tube diameter.
    C. is inversely related to the pressure exerted on the lateral wall.
    D. all of the above.

23. As the temperature increases, the viscosity of a gas _____ and the viscosity of a liquid _____.
    A. becomes lower; becomes higher
    B. becomes higher, becomes lower
    C. becomes lower; stays unchanged
    D. stays unchanged; becomes lower

24. Refer to equation 14-25 in the textbook, the Poiseuille Equation shows that the velocity of a gas is:
    A. directly related to the pressure gradient.
    B. directly related to the fluid viscosity.
    C. directly related to the length of tubing.
    D. inversely related to the fourth power of the radius.

25. Airway resistance is directly related to the _____ and inversely related to the _____.
    A. flow; pressure gradient
    B. flow; elastance
    C. pressure gradient; flow
    D. pressure gradient; elastance

26. To calculate the pulmonary vascular resistance (PVR), the pressure gradient of the pulmonary circulation is expressed as the difference between:
    A. mean pulmonary artery pressure and central venous pressure.
    B. mean pulmonary artery pressure and pulmonary artery wedge pressure.
    C. mean arterial pressure and central venous pressure.
    D. mean arterial pressure and pulmonary artery wedge pressure.

27. To calculate the systemic vascular resistance (SVR), the pressure gradient of the systemic circulation is expressed as the difference between:
    A. mean pulmonary artery pressure and central venous pressure.
    B. mean pulmonary artery pressure and pulmonary artery wedge pressure.
    C. mean arterial pressure and central venous pressure.
    D. mean arterial pressure and pulmonary artery wedge pressure.

28. Rotating vane anemometer, hot wire anemometer, and pneumotachometer are some devices that can be used to measure:
    A. oxygen concentration.
    B. viscosity.
    C. pressure.
    D. volume or flow.

29. _____ is used to describe the volume of gas remaining in the lungs and it is the _____ of resistance and compliance.
    A. Time constant; sum
    B. Time constant; product
    C. Equation of motion; sum
    D. Equation of motion; product

30. Thermodilution is a technique based on the _____ principle to measure a person's _____.
    A. Bernoulli; heat exchange
    B. Bernoulli; cardiac output
    C. Fick; heat exchange
    D. Fick; cardiac output

CHAPTER 15

Chemistry for Respiratory Care

1. The element oxygen (O) has an atomic number of _____ because it has _____.
   A. 8; 8 protons
   B. 16; 16 electrons
   C. 16; 16 protons
   D. 32; 16 electrons

2. Since the atomic number and atomic weight for potassium (K) are 19 and 39 respectively, K has:
   A. 20 protons.
   B. 20 neutrons.
   C. 20 electrons.
   D. all of the above.

3. Atoms with nuclei that have the same number of protons but a different number of neutrons are called:
   A. elements.
   B. compounds.
   C. molecules.
   D. isotopes.

4. The most abundant element in a human body is:
   A. hydrogen.
   B. carbon.
   C. oxygen.
   D. nitrogen.

5. The primary difference between ionic and covalent bonds is the way _____ are used.
   A. electrolytes
   B. electrons
   C. anions
   D. atoms

6. The element sodium carries a _____ charge and this characteristic makes sodium a(n) _____.
   A. positive, cation
   B. positive; anion
   C. negative, cation
   D. negative; anion

7. The chemical reaction $CO_2 + H_2O \; H_2CO_3$ is a(n) _____ reaction.
   A. exchange
   B. decomposition
   C. acidic
   D. synthesis

8. The solubility of a solute is directly related to all of the following conditions *except*:
   A. surface area.
   B. temperature.
   C. pressure.
   D. concentration of solution.

9. A patient asks you about the concentration of a 10% Mucomyst solution. You would explain to the patient that this solution has _____ of active ingredient dissolved in _____ mL of solution.
   A. 1 g or 1,000 mg; 100
   B. 1 g or 10,000 mg; 1,000
   C. 10 g or 10,000 mg; 100
   D. 10 g or 1,000 mg; 10

10. Which of the following solutions has the highest osmotic pressure?
    A. water
    B. 0.45% NaCl
    C. 0.9% NaCl
    D. 1.8% NaCl

11. When a large volume of 0.1% NaCl solution is rapidly administered into the body, the cells would _____ because the solution is _____ relative to the body fluid.
    A. swell; hypertonic
    B. swell; hypotonic
    C. shrink; hypertonic
    D. shrink; hypotonic

12. In addition to water, all of the following are inorganic molecules or compounds *except*:
    A. electrolytes.
    B. carbohydrates.
    C. oxygen.
    D. carbon dioxide.

13. The pH value reflects the _____ concentration in a solution. A high concentration would lead to a _____ pH.
    A. carbon dioxide; high
    B. carbon dioxide; low
    C. hydrogen ion; high
    D. hydrogen ion; low

14. As you are reviewing a patient's medical history, you notice that the pH of two consecutive blood gases drops from 7.00 to 6.00. This means the number of _____ in the arterial blood has _____ by 10 times.
    A. hydrogen ions; increased
    B. hydrogen ions; decreased
    C. cations; increased
    D. cations; decreased

15. The primary function of a buffer in the blood is to maintain a relatively stable:
    A. cardiac output.
    B. pH.
    C. body temperature.
    D. electrolyte level.

16. A salt results when:
    A. acid is added to water.
    B. acid is added to base.
    C. base is added to water.
    D. all of the above.

17. Carbohydrate molecules contain all of the following elements *except*:
    A. nitrogen.
    B. carbon.
    C. oxygen.
    D. hydrogen.

18. Carbohydrates:
    A. do not contain the element oxygen.
    B. use glucose as the building block.
    C. cannot be stored when in excess.
    D. all of the above.

Questions 19 to 22: Match the types of protein in Column I with the respective primary functions in Column II. Use each answer ONCE.

Column I   Column II

19. Hormone   A. Increases the speed of chemical reaction in the body.
20. Keratin   B. Regulates some chemical processes of the body.
21. Collagen   C. Holds most of the body tissues together.
22. Enzyme   D. Forms a network of waterproof fibers in the outer layer of the skin.

23. Lipids:
    A. are soluble in water.
    B. do not include steroids and prostaglandins.
    C. provide a source of energy for the body.
    D. are composed primarily of nitrogen and phosphorus.

24. _____ are the primary component of pulmonary surfactant, and lack of surfactant tends to _____ the surface tension of the lungs.
    A. Lipids; increase
    B. Lipids; decrease
    C. Phospholipids; increase
    D. Phospholipids; decrease

25. Steroids (e.g., estrogen, testosterone) belong to the _____ group.
    A. protein
    B. lipid
    C. carbohydrate
    D. nucleic acid

Questions 26 to 29: Match the terms related to the nucleotide in Column I with the respective characteristics in Column II. Use each answer ONCE.

Column I   Column II

26. Deoxyribonucleic acid (DNA)   A. Translates the genetic information stored in another nucleic acid into protein structures.
27. Ribonucleic acid (RNA)   B. Relaxes the smooth muscles of the airways.
28. Adenosine triphosphate (ATP)   C. Carries the genetic information for the synthesis of proteins.
29. Cyclic 3'5'-adenosine monophosphate (cAMP)   D. Stores energy produced by a nucleotide.

30. Under normal conditions, most fluid loss occurs through the:
    A. skin as perspiration.
    B. lungs as water vapor.
    C. kidneys as urine.
    D. gastrointestinal tract as feces.

31. In two compartments separated by a semipermeable membrane, compartment I is filled with a 10% saline solution and compartment II is filled with a 5% solution. After several hours, you would expect to see the fluid level in:
    A. compartment I to rise.
    B. compartment II to rise.
    C. both compartment to rise.
    D. both compartments to stay the same.

32. The protein concentration in the intravascular compartment is _____ than that in the interstitial compartment, thus generating a(n) _____ pressure to keep the fluid within the intravascular compartment.
    A. higher; osmotic
    B. higher; hydrostatic
    C. lower; osmotic
    D. lower; hydrostatic

33. The hormone aldosterone increases resorption of sodium in the kidney tubule and the result is a(n) _____ in urine volume. This process helps to compensate for systemic _____.
    A. increase; overhydration
    B. increase; dehydration
    C. decrease; overhydration
    D. decrease; dehydration

34. When the blood pressure is low, the _____ in the aortic bodies sends the message to the pituitary gland. In turn, this triggers secretion of antidiuretic hormone and _____ of fluid.
    A. chemoreceptors; retention
    B. chemoreceptors; unloading
    C. baroreceptors; retention
    D. baroreceptors; unloading

Questions 35 to 37: Match the causes of edema in Column I with the respective etiologies in Column II. Use each answer ONCE.

Column I   Column II

35. Retention of excessive electrolytes in the extracellular fluid

36. An increase in capillary hydrostatic pressure

37. A decrease in plasma proteins because of overall protein depletion

A. Poor nutrition as reflected in a low serum albumin level or increased capillary permeability

B. Increased aldosterone secretion or after severe renal disease

C. Congestive heart failure

38. In reviewing a patient's chart, you find that some electrolyte values are as follows: Na^+ = 152 mEq/L, K^+ = 4 mEq/L, Cl^- = 101 mEq/L. You would interpret this finding as:
    A. normal.
    B. hypernatremia.
    C. hypokalemia.
    D. hyperchloremia.

39. Carbonate anhydrase is an enzyme _____ the red blood cells and its primary function is to speed up the reaction of water and carbon dioxide to form _____.
    A. inside; carbonic acid
    B. inside; bicarbonate
    C. outside; carbonic acid
    D. outside; bicarbonate

40. A student asks you to describe the factors leading to a normal pH. You would explain to him that 7.40 (the normal arterial pH) results when the _____ ratio is 20 to 1.
    A. PCO_2 to bicarbonate
    B. carbonic acid to bicarbonate
    C. bicarbonate to PCO_2
    D. bicarbonate to carbonic acid

41. A physician asks you to assess the patient's level of alveolar ventilation. You would evaluate the patient's arterial:
    A. pH.
    B. PO_2.
    C. PCO_2.
    D. HCO_3^-.

42. In the Henderson-Hasselbalch (pH) equation, the carbonic acid level may be calculated as:
    A. PCO_2 x 0.3.
    B. PCO_2 x 0.03.
    C. PCO_2 x 0.003
    D. PCO_2/0.003.

43. In hypoventilation, the _____ cross the gas-permeable blood-brain barrier and _____ the pH of the cerebrospinal fluid. This in turns triggers the medullary center to cause the respiratory muscles to breathe deeper and faster.
    A. CO_2 molecules; increase
    B. CO_2 molecules; decrease
    C. H^+ ions; increase
    D. H^+ ions; increase

44. _____ is a decomposition process involving the oxidation of nutrient molecules. It releases energy as heat and end products including lactic acid, ethanol, CO_2, urea, ammonia, and water.
    A. Metabolism
    B. Anabolism
    C. Catabolism
    D. All of the above

Questions 45 to 47: Match the stages of catabolism in Column I with the respective processes in Column II. Use each answer ONCE.

Column I   Column II

45. Stage 1   A. Goes into citric acid cycle and oxidative phosphorylation to give CO_2, water, and
46. Stage 2   ATP molecules
               B. Breaks down the proteins, carbohydrates
47. Stage 3   (polysaccharides), and lipids (fats) into their respective building blocks
               C. Converts amino acids, glucose, fatty acids, and glycerol into simpler by-products and eventual pyruvic acid and acetyl-CoA or lactic acid

48. The citric acid (Kreb) cycle takes place in the mitochondria of the cell in the presence of _____ and it converts two _____ molecules into six CO_2 and six H_2O molecules.
    A. oxygen; pyruvic acid
    B. oxygen; citric acid
    C. nitrogen; pyruvic acid
    D. nitrogen; citric acid

49. During a metabolic study, you notice the patient's CO_2 production is increased. You may link this observation to all of the following conditions *except*:
    A. hypothermia
    B. exercise
    C. sepsis
    D. severe burns

50. In the body, CO_2 exists in all of the following forms *except*:
    A. dissolved in plasma (about 8% of the total CO_2).
    B. combined with carbamino compounds (about 12% of the total CO_2).
    C. carried as bicarbonate (about 80% of the total CO_2).
    D. transformed into carbon monoxide (less than 0.1% of the total CO_2).

Questions 51 to 53: Mr. Jones, a patient with severe anemia, is admitted to the medical floor for further workup. The following data are gathered from his laboratory reports: Hb = 7 g/100 mL; SaO_2 = 80%; PaO_2 = 70 mm Hg.

51. The amount of dissolved oxygen is:
    A. 0.21 vol%.
    B. 0.7 vol%.
    C. 2.1 vol%.
    D. 5.6 vol%.

52. The amount of oxygen that is attached to the hemoglobin is:
    A. 0.7 vol%.
    B. 5.6 vol%.
    C. 7.5 vol%.
    D. 10.7 vol%.

53. The arterial oxygen content is:
    A. 0.91 vol%.
    B. 7.7 vol%.
    C. 8.7 vol%.
    D. 10.9 vol%.

54. During oxygen rounds, you obtained from the patient a SpO_2 reading of 90%. If the SpO_2 correlates closely with the actual SaO_2, the patient's expected PaO_2 would be about:
    A. 60 mm Hg.
    B. 70 mm Hg.
    C. 80 mm Hg.
    D. 90 mm Hg.

CHAPTER 16 Respiratory Microbiology, Infection, and Infection Control

1. Anaerobic bacteria are _____ organisms that have very _____ oxygen requirement for growth and reproduction.
   A. single-celled; high
   B. multi-celled; high
   C. single-celled; low
   D. multi-celled; low

2. In reviewing a patient's chart, you notice that the sputum sample shows gram-positive microbes. You would infer that the sample had a _____ color after the staining procedure.
   A. violet
   B. pink
   C. white
   D. brown

3. Bacteria become antibiotic-resistant by altering the _____ traits via mutation, conjugation, or transduction.
   A. infection
   B. chemical
   C. metabolic
   D. genetic

4. Bacteria reproduce by the process of _____ and the most rapid phase of reproduction is called the

   _____.
   A. cellular division; log phase
   B. cellular division; lag phase
   C. binary fission; log phase
   D. binary fission; lag phase

5. Food poisoning is caused by the _____ produced by the bacteria and it _____ necessary for the bacteria to be present during this mechanism of disease formation.
   A. toxin; is
   B. toxin; is not
   C. tissue damage; is
   D. tissue damage, is not

Questions 6 to 8: Match the terms in Column I with the descriptions in Column II. Use each answer ONCE.

Column I

6. Nosocomial infection

7. Normal flora

8. Community-acquired pneumonia

Column II

A. The resident bacteria that are harmless at the site.
B. The infection that is acquired outside a health care setting.
C. The infection that is acquired in the hospital.

9. In culture and sensitivity test, *culture* refers to the _____ of pathogenic microbes, and *sensitivity* is done to identify the type and effectiveness of _____ for this particular infection.
   A. identification; antibiotics
   B. identification; treatments
   C. disease resistance; antibiotics
   D. disease resistance; treatments

10. *Chlamydiae* are _____ growing only _____ host cells.
   A. fungi, inside
   B. fungi, outside
   C. bacteria, inside
   D. bacteria, outside

11. *Chlamydiae* are generally infections carried by _____ vectors and they are responsible for atypical pneumonias such as Chlamydia pneumonia and psittacosis.
   A. human
   B. airborne
   C. insect
   D. secretion

12. *Rickettsiae* are _____ and they are generally transmitted to human by _____ vectors. Q fever is an exception where the microbes (*Rickettsia burnetti*) are transmitted by airborne vectors.
    A. viruses; insect
    B. viruses; human
    C. bacteria; insect
    D. bacteria; human

13. Mycoplasmas are free-living _____ and they are responsible for most pneumonias in _____.
    A. bacteria; children and young adults
    B. mycobacteria; old and immunocompromised patients
    C. viruses; children and young adults
    D. fungi; old and immunocompromised patients

14. All of the following terms are related to *Mycobacterium tuberculosis except*:
    A. purified protein derivative.
    B. acid-fast bacilli.
    C. aerobe.
    D. gram-positive bacteria.

15. A patient tells you that he has tested positive for PPD skin test. Based on this information, you may conclude that the patient:
    A. has active pulmonary tuberculosis.
    B. has been exposed to mycobacteria in the past.
    C. should be retested with PPD.
    D. no longer has pulmonary tuberculosis.

16. Viruses are responsible for all of the following infections *except*:
    A. influenza and upper respiratory infections.
    B. chicken pox and infant bronchiolitis.
    C. candidiasis and aspergillosis.
    D. measles and yellow fever.

17. Fungal infections may be transmitted by all of the following methods *except*:
    A. inhalation of dust.
    B. skin-to-skin contact.
    C. insect bites.
    D. inhalation of dried bird droppings.

18. *Pneumocystis carinii* has been classified as a _____ and it is responsible for the development of _____ in immunocompromised patients.
    A. virus; pneumocystis pneumonia
    B. fungus; pneumocystis pneumonia
    C. virus; tuberculosis
    D. fungus; tuberculosis

19. A parasite is a _____ that lives on a host.
    A. virus
    B. fungus
    C. plant
    D. plant or animal

20. One of the most serious concerns in the use of antibiotics is that:
    A. antibiotics are expensive.
    B. antibiotics are hard to administer.
    C. bacteria are rapidly developing resistance to antibiotics.
    D. insurance reimbursement rate for antibiotics is low.

21. MRSA and VRE are both _____ highly resistant to most _____.
    A. viruses; sterilization procedures
    B. bacteria; sterilization procedures
    C. viruses; antibiotics
    D. bacteria; antibiotics

22. Critical equipment and supplies such as chest tubes must be _____, which means _____ of all organisms.
    A. disinfected; reducing the number
    B. sterilized; complete killing
    C. disinfected; complete killing
    D. sterilized; reducing the number

23. A classmate asks you about the sterilization procedure suitable for equipment that cannot withstand high temperatures or immersion in fluid. You would suggest:
    A. ethylene oxide.
    B. Cidex.
    C. QUAT.
    D. 70% alcohol.

24. The department manager asks you to write up a set of guidelines to ensure sterility of RT equipment. You would include in the guidelines the use of:
    A. indicator tape during sterilization.
    B. temperature and pressure recordings.
    C. culture samples from equipment.
    D. expiration date of chemicals.

25. Universal precautions are required when contact with _____ is likely.
    A. blood
    B. tears
    C. sputum
    D. body fluids

26. _____ is the most effective way to limit the incidence of cross-contamination.
    A. Hand washing
    B. Isolation
    C. Reverse isolation
    D. Wearing gloves and gown

27. All of the following conditions are considered upper respiratory infections *except*:
    A. epiglottitis.
    B. pneumonia.
    C. otitis.
    D. parapharyngeal abscess.

28. After an outbreak of infection in the ICU, you are trying to determine if the source of infection originated from the RT department. Which of the following RT equipment and supplies is *least* likely the source of nosocomial infections?
    A. Mechanical ventilators
    B. Heat and moisture exchangers (HMEs)
    C. Use of nonsterile water
    D. Nebulizers

29. Protected brush catheter, bronchoalveolar lavage, and lung biopsy are techniques used to collect _____ via a _____.
    A. sputum samples; suction catheter
    B. sputum samples; flexible bronchoscopy
    C. fluid, cell and tissue samples; suction catheter
    D. fluid, cell and tissue samples; flexible bronchoscopy

30. An ideal sputum sample should be:
    A. collected and kept in a sterile container.
    B. analyzed without delay.
    C. free from contamination by oral secretions.
    D. all of the above.

CHAPTER 17

Cardiopulmonary Anatomy and Physiology

1. In addition to providing gas exchange and acid-base regulation, the respiratory system is capable of:
   A. producing and metabolizing chemicals.
   B. humidifying and conditioning inspired air.
   C. containing pollutants and microbes.
   D. all of the above.

2. When the _____ muscles fail to maintain the proper tone and stability, obstructive sleep apnea may result.
   A. pharyngeal
   B. tracheal
   C. laryngeal
   D. nasal

3. Opening and closing of the glottis, swallowing, coughing, sneezing, and changes in the vocal cords while producing sounds are the functions of the _____ muscles.
   A. nasal
   B. laryngeal
   C. pharyngeal
   D. tracheal

4. Extrinsic laryngeal muscles and sternocleidomastoid muscles are two groups of respiratory muscles that are located _____ the thoracic cavity and they may be used during _____ maneuvers.
   A. within; forced inspiratory
   B. within; forced expiratory
   C. outside; forced inspiratory
   D. outside; forced expiratory

5. There are _____ pairs of ribs and the first _____ pairs attach their anterior portions to the manubrium and body of sternum.
   A. 10; 6
   B. 11; 6
   C. 12; 7
   D. 12; 7

Questions 6 to 10: Match the respiratory muscles within the thoracic cavity in Column I with the respective functions in Column II. Use each answer ONCE.

Column I

6. Diaphragm

7. External intercostal and parasternal portion of internal intercostal muscles

8. Lateral portion of internal intercostal and vertebrocostal muscles

9. Pectoralis minor and major, serratus anterior, and erector spinae

10. Abdominal muscles (rectus abdominis, external and internal oblique and transversus abdominis)

Column II

A. Raise the ribs, push the sternum forward and upward, and straighten the concavity of the thoracic spine
B. Active expiration
C. Normal continuous respiration and other non-ventilatory functions such as labor, vomiting, and defecation
D. Depress the lower ribs, increase intra-abdominal pressure, and flex the thoracic spine
E. Active inspiration

11. The right lung has _____ lobes and _____ segments.
    A. 2; 7
    B. 2; 8
    C. 3; 9
    D. 3; 10

12. Inferior and superior lingular segments are part of the:
    A. left upper lobe.
    B. left lower lobe.
    C. right upper lobe.
    D. right middle lobe.

13. Gas exchange takes place at the level of:
    A. alveoli.
    B. alveolar sacs.
    C. respiratory bronchioles.
    D. all of the above.

14. Select the proper sequence of pulmonary blood flow. (Note: not all structures are listed.)
    A. Right ventricle, pulmonary veins, pulmonary arteries, left atrium
    B. Right ventricle, pulmonary arteries, pulmonary veins, left atrium
    C. Left ventricle, pulmonary veins, pulmonary arteries, right atrium
    D. Right ventricle, pulmonary arteries, pulmonary veins, left atrium

15. Blood supply to the tracheobronchial tree, hilar lymph nodes, visceral pleura, pulmonary arteries and veins, vagus nerve, and esophagus are provided by the _____ circulation.
    A. pulmonary
    B. coronary
    C. bronchial
    D. lymphatic

16. The primary function of the lymphatic system is to:
    A. provide fluid and electrolyte balance.
    B. prevent infection of the lungs.
    C. provide adequate blood flow to the tracheobronchial tree.
    D. prevent accumulation of fluid in the alveoli.

Questions 17 to 19: Match the receptors of the pulmonary system in Column I with the locations in Column II. Use ONLY THREE answers.

Column I

17. Irritant receptors
18. Stretch receptors
19. C-fiber or J-type receptors

Column II

A. Alveolar walls, airways, and pulmonary blood vessels
B. Epithelium of extrapulmonary airways
C. Nasopharynx
D. Trachea and main stem bronchi
E. Smooth muscles of the lungs

Questions 20 to 22: Match the receptors of the pulmonary system in Column I with the respective triggers and responses in Column II. Use each answer ONCE.

Column I

20. Irritant receptors
21. Stretch receptors
22. C-fiber or J-type receptors

Column II

A. In response to lung inflation or increased transpulmonary pressure causing bronchodilation, increase in heart rate, and decreased peripheral systemic vascular resistance
B. In response to increased interstitial congestion, chemical injury, or microemboli by initiating a rapid, shallow breathing pattern, bronchoconstriction, bradycardia, and increased mucus secretion
C. In response to smoke or foreign particles leading to bronchoconstriction, increased ventilation, constriction of the larynx, cough, and increased mucus secretion

23. Visceral pleura is the lining that covers the _____ and parietal pleura covers the inside of the _____.
    A. lung, chest wall
    B. lung, mediastinum
    C. chest wall, lung
    D. mediastinum, lung

24. Excessive fluid in the pleural space is removed by the:
    A. cilia.
    B. pulmonary perfusion.
    C. lungs.
    D. lymphatic vessels.

25. All structures within the thorax except the lungs and pleurae are contained within the:
    A. chest wall.
    B. mediastinum.
    C. thoracic cavity.
    D. abdominal cavity.

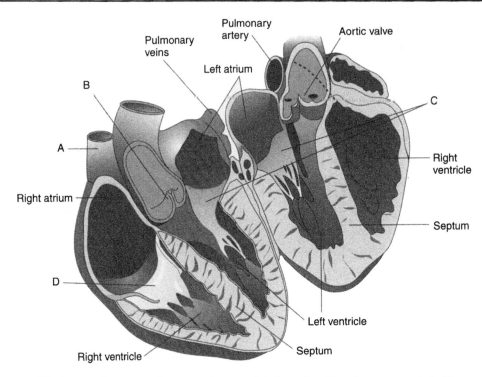

The heart and great vessels presented in a medial plane that slices the structures in half.

26. Referring to the figure shown above, _____ represents the tricuspid valve and it is open during _____.
    A. A; systole
    B. B; diastole
    C. C; systole
    D. D; diastole

27. Select the proper sequence of blood flow through the heart. (Note: not all structures are listed.)
    A. Right atrium, right ventricle, tricuspid valve, left atrium
    B. Right atrium, tricuspid valve, mitral valve, left ventricle
    C. Right ventricle, pulmonic valve, aortic valve, left atrium
    D. Right ventricle, left atrium, aortic valve, left ventricle

28. Select the proper sequence of cardiac electrical conduction. (Note: not all structures are listed.)
    A. AV node, SA node, bundle of His, bundle branches
    B. AV node, bundle of His, Purkinje fibers, bundle branches
    C. SA node, AV node, Purkinje fibers, bundle of His
    D. SA node, AV node, bundle of His, bundle branches

29. The blood supply to the coronary circulation of the heart arises from the:
    A. ascending aorta, and right and left aortic sinuses.
    B. ascending aorta and left aortic sinus.
    C. descending aorta and right aortic sinus.
    D. descending aorta and left aortic sinus.

30. The functions of the mucociliary apparatus may be impaired by:
    A. chronic lung disorder.
    B. viral infection.
    C. prolonged intubation.
    D. all of the above.

31. Arterial blood gases done on a patient reveal acidosis (low pH), hypercapnia (high PCO_2), and hypoxemia (low PO_2). These findings may cause _____ due to the direct effect on the _____.
    A. bronchodilation; smooth muscle cells
    B. bronchodilation; parasympathetic branches
    C. bronchoconstriction; smooth muscle cells
    D. bronchoconstriction; sympathetic branches

32. Neutralizing and eliminating inhaled agents that may be harmful to the lung is the primary function of:
    A. macrophages.
    B. cilia.
    C. dendritic cells.
    D. mast cells.

33. Type II alveolar cells are responsible for the:
    A. production, secretion, and clearance of surfactant.
    B. clearance of excess alveolar fluid.
    C. reduction of work of breathing.
    D. all of the above.

34. Following lung injury, an increased level of _____ may lead to formation of lung fibrosis.
    A. macrophages
    B. fibronectin
    C. alveolar type I cells
    D. mast cells

35. During normal tidal inspiration, the pressure in the lungs is _____ the pressure at the mouth or nose opening.
    A. higher than
    B. lower than
    C. equal to
    D. 10 cm H_2O higher than

36. The work of breathing is usually _____ when the elastic recoil of the lung is high as seen in _____.
    A. decreased; lung fibrosis
    B. decreased; emphysema
    C. increased; lung fibrosis
    D. increased; emphysema

37. A patient has the following measurements during spontaneous breathing: volume change = 0.4 L; pressure change = 4 cm H_2O. The calculated compliance is:
    A. 0.1 L/cm H_2O.
    B. 1 L/cm H_2O.
    C. 1 cm H_2O/L.
    D. 10 cm H_2O/L.

38. Since airway resistance is inversely proportional to the _____ power of the radius, decrease of the airway radius by 50% would increase the resistance by _____ times.
    A. 4th; 8
    B. 4th; 16
    C. 2nd; 4
    D. 2nd; 8

39. One of the methods to evaluate a patient's endurance of respiratory muscles is to measure the:
    A. tidal volume.
    B. vital capacity.
    C. maximal voluntary ventilation.
    D. peak flow.

40. Alveolar dead space is the lung volume that cannot take part in gas exchange due to lack of _____. An example is _____.
    A. pulmonary perfusion; pulmonary embolism
    B. pulmonary perfusion; emphysema
    C. ventilation; pulmonary embolism
    D. ventilation; emphysema

41. Blood flow to the lungs is influenced by:
    A. gravity.
    B. hypoxia.
    C. hypercapnia.
    D. all of the above.

42. Hypoxemia (low PO_2) general occurs _____ hypercapnia (high PCO_2) because _____ has a higher solubility and a smaller pressure gradient between the venous blood and alveolar gas.
    A. before; CO_2
    B. before; O_2
    C. after; CO_2
    D. after; O_2

43. Due to its high affinity to _____, carbon monoxide is useful in testing the _____ across the lungs.
    A. plasma; diffusion capacity
    B. plasma; gas solubility
    C. hemoglobin; diffusion capacity
    D. hemoglobin; gas solubility

CHAPTER **18**

Respiratory Pharmacology

1. Levalbuterol is a stereoisomer of _____ that rotates the light to the _____. This stereoisomer provides optimal therapeutic effects while eliminating the unwanted side effects.
   A. albuterol; left
   B. albuterol; right
   C. racemic epinephrine; left
   D. racemic epinephrine; right

2. Since many drugs are weak acids or bases, they become _____ easily and unable to move across the

   _____.
   A. bonded; lipid cell membranes
   B. bonded; interstitial space
   C. ionized; lipid cell membranes
   D. ionized; interstitial space

3. For maximal drug deposition to the lower airways, the ideal size of aerosol particles should be smaller than:
   A. 1 micron.
   B. 3 microns.
   C. 5 microns.
   D. 10 microns.

4. Drugs given by aerosol to the lower airways have less than _____ deposition and near _____ absorption of the administered dose.
   A. 20%; 70%
   B. 20%; 100%
   C. 50%; 50%
   D. 50%; 70%

5. Rank the following routes of drug administration in the order of systemic absorption (from fastest to slowest absorption).
   A. Intravenous, intramuscular, aerosol, oral
   B. Intramuscular, aerosol, oral, intravenous
   C. Oral, aerosol, intervenous, intramuscular
   D. Aerosol, intravenous, intramuscular, oral

6. Volume of drug distribution is determined by the:
   A. amount of the drug in the body.
   B. plasma concentration of the drug.
   C. drug dosage in a 24-hour period.
   D. A and B only.

7. Drugs may be cleared from the body by:
   A. biotransformation.
   B. elimination.
   C. molecular diffusion.
   D. A and B.

8. Drugs that have undergone biotransformation are called _____ and they may stay active, become inactive, or develop _____ effects.
   A. stereoisomers; toxic
   B. stereoisomers; sedative
   C. metabolites; toxic
   D. metabolites; sedative

9. To determine the speed of drug elimination by the _____, _____ is used as a marker.
   A. kidneys; creatinine
   B. kidneys; P-450 enzyme
   C. liver; creatinine
   D. liver; P-450 enzyme

10. _____ refers to the time that is required for the body, tissue, or organ to metabolize or inactivate half of the administered drug dosage.
    A. Elimination factor
    B. Half-life
    C. Clearance factor
    D. Absorption coefficient

11. A drug that stimulates a receptor site is called a(n):
    A. agonist.
    B. antagonist.
    C. stimulator.
    D. activator.

12. The type of drug receptors that provides the quickest mechanism by which the drug's effect is achieved is the _____ receptors.
    A. tyrosine kinase-linked
    B. G protein-coupled
    C. ligand-gated channel
    D. steroid

13. The degree of drug binding and unbinding to a receptor depends on:
    A. drug concentration.
    B. affinity of the drug to the receptor.
    C. dissociation constant.
    D. all of the above.

14. _____ refers to the maximum achievable effect that a drug is able to produce.
    A. Potency
    B. Efficacy
    C. Concentration
    D. Maximum effective dose

15. Off-label use of a prescription drug is:
    A. approved by the Food and Drug Administration (FDA).
    B. based on the indication for which a drug is given.
    C. based on additional indications other than those approved by the FDA.
    D. illegal in the United States.

16. _____ is a condition in which the dosage must be increased over time in order to achieve the same effect.
    A. Tolerance
    B. Toxicity
    C. Contraindication
    D. Side effect

17. Type _____ intermediate hypersensitivity is mediated by immunoglobulin E (IgE) class antibodies and this reaction involves eventual degranulation of the mast cells.
    A. I
    B. II
    C. III
    D. IV

18. _____ can be found in the _____ and they are capable of recruiting other inflammatory cells such as neutrophils and lymphocytes.
    A. Mast cells; lungs
    B. Macrophages; airways
    C. Mast cells and macrophages; airways
    D. Mast cells and macrophages; lungs

19. The first step in the induction of inflammation is the presence of a(n):
    A. antibody.
    B. antigen.
    C. histamine.
    D. cytokines.

Questions 20 to 23: Match the types of mediators in Column I with the respective actions on the airway in Column II. Use each answer ONCE.

Column I

20. Adrenergic system
21. Cholinergic system
22. Leukotrienes (slow-reacting substance of anaphylaxis)
23. Histamine

Column II

A. Direct effects on bronchial and vascular smooth muscle, causing contraction
B. Stimulation of β-2 receptors, causing relaxation of smooth muscle
C. Vagal stimulation of M_3 muscarinic receptors, causing smooth muscle contraction and bronchoconstriction
D. Direct action on smooth muscle cells through their own receptor, causing tonic bronchoconstriction

Questions 24 to 27: Match the types of mediators in Column I with the respective actions on the bronchial secretions in Column II. Use each answer ONCE.

Column I

24. Adrenergic system
25. Cholinergic system
26. Histamine
27. Inflammation

Column II

A. Production of secretions in the upper and lower airways and increasing vascular permeability, leading to edema
B. Production of bronchial secretions and stimulation of cholinergic responses
C. Enhancement of mucociliary clearance in the bronchi and fluid clearance from the alveoli
D. Stimulation of bronchial goblet cells and production of mucus by means of M_3 receptors

28. Relaxation of the bronchial smooth muscles is a desirable effect of _____ adrenergic receptors.
    A. alpha
    B. β-1
    C. β-2
    D. omega

29. Dr. Abel tells you that her patient has developed side effects from prolonged use and absorption of adrenergic agonists. These side effects may include all of the following *except*:
    A. palpitations.
    B. tremor.
    C. bradycardia.
    D. hypertension.

30. Cholinergic antagonists are also called _____ agents and they cause _____.
    A. anticholinergic; bronchodilation
    B. anticholinergic; bronchoconstriction
    C. histaminergic; bronchodilation
    D. histaminergic; bronchoconstriction

31. When respiratory drugs are given via the inhalation route, the main disadvantage is that the volume of drug delivered is:
    A. absorbed too fast.
    B. poorly absorbed.
    C. highly variable due to external factors.
    D. diluted too much.

32. In order to achieve maximum bronchodilation with minimal side effects, the respiratory drug should be long-lasting and highly selective in _____ activity. An example of this drug is _____.
    A. β-1; norepinephrine
    B. β-1; albuterol
    C. β-2; terbutaline
    D. β-2; salmeterol

Questions 33 to 39: Match the dosing abbreviations in Column I with the respective meanings in Column II. Use each answer ONCE.

Column I   Column II

33. PO   A. Every four hours
            B. Under the tongue
34. IV   C. As needed
            D. To be given via the vein
35. SC   E. Four times daily
            F. To be given by mouth
36. SL   G. Under the skin

37. q4h

38. qid

39. prn

40. Atropine is an example of _____ drugs that block the stimulation of the _____ receptors, thus promoting bronchodilation.
    A. anticholinergic; cholinergic
    B. anticholinergic; adrenergic
    C. cholinergic; vagal
    D. cholinergic; β-1

41. The likely mechanism of action for methylxanthines is _____ and _____ is an example of this class of drugs.
    A. excitation of phosphodiesterase; epinephrine
    B. inhibition of phosphodiesterase; theophylline
    C. excitation of β-2 receptors; albuterol
    D. inhibition of β-1 receptors; Atrovent

Questions 42 to 45: Match the types of bronchodilators in Column I with the examples in Column II. Use each answer ONCE.

Column I   Column II

42. Short-acting β-2 agonist   A. Albuterol
                                  B. Theophylline
43. Long-acting β-agonist   C. Salmeterol
                                  D. Ipratropium
44. Anticholinergic

45. Methylxanthine

46. In prolonged or high-dose use of systemic _____, sodium retention, edema, and hypertension are some complications.
    A. antibiotics
    B. cromones
    C. bronchodilators
    D. steroids

47. When inhaled steroids are used to treat acute exacerbation of asthma, a short-acting bronchodilator is recommended. This is because:
    A. bronchodilators are more effective than steroids.
    B. the steroids may not work.
    C. of the delayed onset of inhaled steroids.
    D. bronchodilators are easier to administer.

48. To minimize the occurrence of thrush, the patient should _____ following use of _____.
    A. rinse the mouth; glucocorticoid
    B. rinse the mouth; inhaled beclomethasone
    C. use an MDI bronchodilator; mineralocorticoid
    D. use an MDI bronchodilator; inhaled dexamethasone

49. Acetylsalicylic acid is the generic name for _____ and it is classified as a _____.
    A. aspirin; steroidal antiinflammatory drug (SAID)
    B. dexamethasone; steroidal antiinflammatory drug (SAID)
    C. aspirin; nonsteroidal antiinflammatory drug (NSAID)
    D. dexamethasone; steroidal antiinflammatory drug (NSAID)

50. _____, originally described as SRS-A (slow-reacting substance of anaphylaxis), is a substance that causes prolonged smooth muscle contraction, bronchospasm, and inflammation.
    A. Histamine
    B. Leukotriene
    C. Cromone
    D. Xanthine

51. Cromones are classified as _____ drugs and they are used for the _____ management of mild asthma and exercise-induced bronchospasm.
    A. steroidal; acute
    B. steroidal; prophylactic
    C. antiinflammatory; acute
    D. antiinflammatory; prophylactic

52. Benadryl, Claritin, Allegra, and Zyrtec are classified as:
    A. antihistamines.
    B. steroidal agents.
    C. antiinflammatory drugs.
    D. bronchodilators.

53. N-acetyl-L-cysteine or acetylcysteine is a _____ agent. It should be given with a prophylactic dose of bronchodilator because acetylcysteine tends to induce _____ when used alone.
    A. bronchoconstrictive; bronchospasm
    B. bronchoconstrictive; productive coughs
    C. mucolytic; bronchospasm
    D. mucolytic; productive coughs

54. Exosurf, Survanta, and Infasurf are drugs used to _____ the surface tension of the lungs of _____ neonates.
    A. increase; post-term
    B. increase; premature
    C. decrease; post-term
    D. decrease; premature

Questions 55 to 59: Match the inhaled antimicrobial drugs in Column I with the common microbial applications in Column II. Use each answer ONCE.

Column I   Column II

55. Ribavirin   A. *Pseudomonas aeruginosa*
                         B. Gram-negative infection
56. Amphotericin B   C. *Pneumocystis carinii* infection
                         D. Pulmonary aspergillosis
57. Tobramycin   E. Respiratory syncytial virus

58. Gentamicin

59. Pentamidine

60. _____ may be used to help stop excessive airway bleeding because it is a(n) _____.
    A. Thrombin; coagulant
    B. Heparin; anticoagulant
    C. Streptokinase; coagulant
    D. Warfarin; anticoagulant

Questions 61 to 65: Match the classes of diuretics in Column I with the respective actions in Column II. Use each answer ONCE.

Column I   Column II

61. Furosemide (Lasix)   A. Blocks sodium resorption and potassium excretion in the distal tubule
62. Hydrochlorothiazide (Esidrix)   B. Blocks resorption of sodium in the ascending loop of Henle
63. Spironolactone (Aldactone)   C. Raises the osmolarity of the urine, pulling in water, and is then excreted
64. Acetazolamide (Diamox)   D. Blocks carbonic anhydrase that interconverts bicarbonate and carbon dioxide in the proximal convoluted tubule
65. Mannitol   E. Blocks sodium permeability of the collecting duct

66. With the *exception* of _____, all other diuretics in questions 61 to 65 above can cause metabolic _____ with hypochloremia.
    A. mannitol; acidosis
    B. Diamox; alkalosis
    C. Lasix; acidosis
    D. Aldactone; alkalosis

67. Epinephrine and dopamine are examples of _____ and they tend to _____ blood pressure and vascular resistance to blood flow.
    A. vasopressors; increase
    B. vasopressors; decrease
    C. vasodilators; increase
    D. vasodilators; decrease

68. Nitroglycerin and nitroprusside help to relieve angina because they are _____ and tend to _____ high blood pressure and vascular resistance to blood flow.
    A. vasopressors; produce
    B. vasopressors; reduce
    C. vasodilators; produce
    D. vasodilators; reduce

69. Stimulation of the mu, delta, or kappa receptors in the brain and spinal cord can significantly reduce the sensation of:
    A. anxiety.
    B. pain.
    C. dyspnea.
    D. hypoxia.

70. Lorazepam (Ativan), diazepam (Valium), propofol (Diprivan) are classified as _____ with different clinical uses.
    A. vasopressors
    B. paralyzing agents
    C. opiates
    D. sedatives

71. Naloxone (Narcan) is used to reverse the effects of:
    A. narcotics.
    B. bronchoconstrictors.
    C. sedatives.
    D. paralyzing agents.

72. Succinylcholine is a _____ neuromuscular blocker as it causes prolonged _____ at the motor endplate, making muscular movement impossible.
    A. depolarizing; depolarization
    B. depolarizing; repolarization
    C. nondepolarizing; depolarization
    D. nondepolarizing; repolarization

73. As a topical drug, the primary clinical application of lidocaine is to anesthetize the larynx and airway prior to:
    A. nasotracheal suctioning.
    B. mechanical ventilation.
    C. bronchoscopy.
    D. sinus surgery.

CHAPTER 19

History and Physical Examination

1. A chronological narrative account of the patient's health problem is called:
   A. activities of daily living (ADL).
   B. history and physical (h & p).
   C. history of present illness (HPI).
   D. vital signs.

2. Mr. Caine, a patient with COPD, has been smoking for 15 years and averaging two packs of cigarettes per day. You would record his smoking history as:
   A. 2 pack years.
   B. 7.5 pack years.
   C. 15 pack years.
   D. 30 pack years.

3. Since cystic fibrosis is a hereditary disease, you would expect to read about it under the _____ section of the patient's medical record.
   A. activities of daily living (ADL)
   B. family history
   C. vital signs
   D. physician's order

4. Under the vital signs section of a patient's medical record, you would find all of the following data except:
   A. heart rate.
   B. systemic blood pressure.
   C. respiratory rate.
   D. blood gas results.

5. From an anterior view of the chest, the _____ is between the left and right clavicles and above the body of sternum.
   A. costal angle
   B. manubrium
   C. thyroid cartilage
   D. xiphoid process

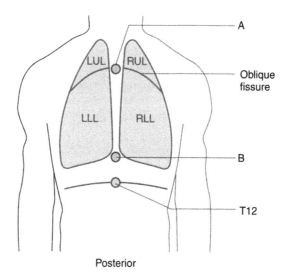

Posterior

Surface anatomy of the posterior thorax.

6. Referring to the figure shown above, the upper and lower borders of the lower lobes (points A and B) are at the _____ levels, respectively.
   A. T2 and T 8
   B. T2 and T10
   C. T3 and T10
   D. T3 and T12

Questions 7 to 10: Match the techniques of assessment in Column I with the respective descriptions in Column II. Use each answer ONCE.

Column I

7. Auscultation
8. Percussion
9. Palpation
10. Inspection

Column II

A. Visually observing the patient
B. Listening to body sounds with a stethoscope placed on the skin surface
C. Placing a finger firmly against a body part and striking that finger with a fingertip from the other hand
D. Using the hands to feel for body movement, lumps, masses, and skin characteristics

Questions 11 to 15: Match the percussion notes in Column I with the respective quality and characteristics in Column II. Use each answer ONCE.

Column I   Column II

11. Flat   A. Medium intensity, pitch, and
                               duration, as elicited by percus-
12. Dull   sion over the liver or a tumor

                            B. Loud and drumlike, with a high
13. Resonant   pitch, as elicited by percussion
                               over a gastric bubble

14. Hyperresonant   C. Very loud, lower in pitch, longer
                               in duration, as elicited by percus-
15. Tympanic   sion over an emphysematous
                               lung or a pneumothorax

                            D. Loud, low in pitch, and of long
                               duration as elicited by percussion
                               over normal lung tissue

                            E. Soft, high-pitched, and of short
                               duration, as elicited by percus-
                               sion of the thigh

16. During shift report, a patient is described to be hypoventilating. This means that the patient:
    A. has a high arterial PCO_2.
    B. has a low arterial PCO_2.
    C. is breathing fast and deep.
    D. is breathing slow and shallow.

17. Ms. Rowland, a patient on the medical floor, has a history of nocturnal orthopnea. This means that she sleeps better in a(n) _____ position.
    A. supine
    B. prone
    C. upright
    D. lateral

18. "Use of accessory muscles" is a term related to all of the following conditions *except:*
    A. retractions.
    B. decreased work of breathing.
    C. more negative intrapleural pressure.
    D. excessive use of neck, back, and abdominal muscles.

19. Nasal flaring is a sign of _____ work of breathing and this breathing technique is used to reduce the _____.
    A. increased; airflow resistance
    B. increased; lung compliance
    C. decreased; airflow resistance
    D. decreased; lung compliance

20. Flail chest usually leads to _____ respiration because the _____ of the chest wall has been compromised.
    A. Cheyne-Stokes; compliance
    B. Kussmaul's; stability
    C. Biot's; compliance
    D. paradoxical; stability

21. A diagnosis of significant left-sided tension pneumothorax has been confirmed on a chest radiograph. From this finding, you would expect to see:
    A. subcutaneous emphysema.
    B. shifting of the trachea to the left.
    C. shifting of the trachea to the right.
    D. clubbing of the digits.

22. Cyanosis is a sign of significant _____ and this bluish hue may be seen in the _____, earlobe, or mucous membrane of the mouth.
    A. desaturation of hemoglobin; nailbeds
    B. desaturation of hemoglobin; eyelids
    C. hypoventilation; nailbeds
    D. hypoventilation; eyelids

23. In the presence of pneumothorax or emphysema, the affected side produces a _____ or tympanic percussion note. This is due to an excessive _____ under the area of percussion.
    A. flat; amount of lung tissue
    B. resonant; volume of air
    C. dull; amount of lung tissue
    D. hyperresonant; air

24. _____ are abnormal breath sounds usually heard at the end of inspiration and are fine quality and high-pitched.
    A. Crackles
    B. Rhonchi
    C. Wheezes
    D. Stridor

25. During physical examination, the physician asks the patient to say the words "ninety nine" while listening to the voice sounds. This technique is called _____ and the spoken words are clearly heard over _____ lungs.
    A. egophony; edematous
    B. whispered pectoriloquy; collapsed
    C. bronchophony; consolidated
    D. bronchial sounds; normal

26. A clinical instructor asks you to locate the topical landmark for the aortic valve. You would point at the _____ interspace to the _____ of the sternal border.
    A. first; left
    B. first; right
    C. second; left
    D. second; right

27. The sternal angle (Angle of Louis) is the joint between the manubrium and sternum. The _____ interspace is located to either side immediately below the sternal angle.
    A. first
    B. second
    C. third
    D. fourth

28. The spinous process of the _____ cervical vertebra may be identified by asking the patient to extend the head and neck forward and down.
    A. fourth
    B. fifth
    C. sixth
    D. seventh

29. The sound of tricuspid valve may be heard at the _____ interspace at the _____ sternal border.
    A. fourth; left
    B. fifth; left
    C. fourth; right
    D. fifth; right

30. As you are reviewing a patient's medical record, you notice that heart murmur is one of the abnormal findings. This condition is usually related to:
    A. regurgitation of blood flow back to the heart chamber.
    B. decrease in cardiac output.
    C. congestive heart failure.
    D. S_3 and S_4 heart sounds.

31. Jugular vein distention suggests congestion or failure of the:
    A. left ventricle.
    B. right ventricle.
    C. pulmonary circulation.
    D. systemic circulation.

32. Glasgow Coma Scale assesses a patient's ability to perform all of the following *except:*
    A. verbal response.
    B. integrated motor response.
    C. respiratory effort.
    D. eye-opening response.

33. A patient is being assessed in the emergency department following a motor vehicle accident. When a painful stimulus is applied, the patient responds with extension and internal rotation of the arms and extends the legs. This is _____ posturing and it indicates a _____.
    A. decerebrate; low-level brain stem compression
    B. decerebrate; lesion in the mesencephalic region of the brain
    C. decorticate; low-level brain stem compression
    D. decorticate; lesion in the mesencephalic region of the brain

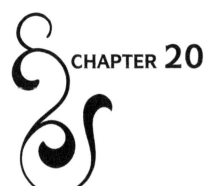

CHAPTER 20

Blood Chemistries and Hematology

1. _____ is the blood component after removal of cells and coagulation proteins.
   A. Platelets
   B. Hemoglobin
   C. Serum
   D. Plasma

2. Electrolytes and other chemistry studies typically measure the quantity of these components in the:
   A. urine.
   B. serum.
   C. red blood cells.
   D. white blood cells.

3. _____ is an anion—an electrolyte that carries a _____ charge.
   A. Phosphate; negative
   B. Sodium; positive
   C. Potassium; positive
   D. Calcium; negative

4. Among the four electrolytes listed below, _____ is the least abundant in the extracellular fluid because 90% of it is intracellular.
   A. Na^+
   B. Cl^-
   C. HCO_3^-
   D. K^+

5. Mr. Jones is admitted to the medical unit for severe dehydration. In reviewing his medical records, you would expect to find all of the following signs of decreased total body water (TBW) *except:*
   A. increased urine output and concentrated urine.
   B. thready rapid pulse.
   C. low blood pressure.
   D. elevated hematocrit, sodium, and protein levels.

6. Ms. Farland, a patient in the SICU, has a serum sodium level of 126 mEq/L and estimated osmolality of 16. Based on these values, the patient's serum sodium level is _____ and her condition may be interpreted as _____.
   A. high; hypernatremia
   B. low; hyponatremia
   C. high; pseudohypernatremia
   D. low; pseudohyponatremia

7. The most recent bloodwork on a patient shows a serum sodium level of 152 mEq/L. This condition may be caused by all of the following *except:*
   A. water loss in excess of sodium loss.
   B. pure water loss.
   C. increase in total body sodium.
   D. hypervolemia secondary to congestive heart failure.

8. Muscular weakness, malaise, fatigue, and myalgia are some neuromuscular signs of:
   A. hypokalemia.
   B. hyperkalemia.
   C. hyponatremia.
   D. hyperchloremia.

9. The laboratory report for Ms. Highland reveals hypokalemia. Her condition may be caused by any of the following conditions *except:*
   A. intracellular shift of potassium due to respiratory or metabolic alkalosis.
   B. acute or chronic renal failure.
   C. use of diuretics such as thiazides and furosemide.
   D. loss of potassium due to vomiting.

10. With the exception of acid-base disturbances, chloride concentration follows changes in serum _____ levels.
    A. magnesium
    B. calcium
    C. sodium
    D. potassium

11. A patient has the following electrolyte measurements: Na^+ = 140 mEq/L; K^+ = 4 mEq/L; Cl^- = 105 mEq/L; CO_2 = 30 mEq/L. The calculated anion gap is _____ and this value shows a(n) _____.
    A. 9 mEq/L; normal anion gap
    B. 35 mEq/L; normal anion gap
    C. 35 mEq/L; elevated anion gap
    D. 110 mEq/L; elevated anion gap

12. Besides being a major structural substance in bone, _____ also maintains cellular conduction in the neuromuscular system and plays a role in the coagulation process.
    A. sodium
    B. magnesium
    C. potassium
    D. calcium

13. Since unbound or _____ calcium is used in clinical practice, its serum measurement should be corrected for the _____ concentration.
    A. charged; albumin
    B. charged; magnesium
    C. ionized; albumin
    D. ionized; magnesium

14. A patient has an ionized calcium level of 8 mg/dL. This condition may be consistent with all of the following clinical signs *except*:
    A. anorexia.
    B. vomiting.
    C. prolonged QT interval in an ECG.
    D. mental confusion.

15. Magnesium is an important electrolyte in maintaining a proper balance of the _____ level.
    A. phosphorus
    B. pH
    C. calcium
    D. potassium

16. Confusion, seizures, coma and osteomalacia may be caused by:
    A. hyperphosphatemia.
    B. hypermagnesemia.
    C. hypophosphatemia.
    D. hypomagnesemia.

17. Since an elevated serum _____ is an important cause of anion gap metabolic acidosis, it is used to evaluate the severity of shock, tissue perfusion, oxygen delivery, and oxygen use.
    A. sodium
    B. bicarbonate
    C. lactate
    D. potassium

Questions 18 to 25: Match the serum electrolytes in Column I with the respective normal ranges in Column II. Use each answer ONCE.

Column I	Column II
18. Sodium (Na^+)	A. 98 to 107 mEq/L
	B. 1.16 to 1.32 mEq/L
19. Potassium (K^+)	C. <2 mEq/L
	D. 1.5 to 2.5 mEq/L
20. Chloride (Cl^-)	E. 0.87 to 1.45 mEq/L
	F. 3.5 to 5.5 mEq/L
21. Carbon dioxide (CO_2)	G. 22 to 32 mEq/L
	H. 135 to 145 mEq/L
22. Ionized calcium (Ca^{+2})	
23. Magnesium (Mg^{+2})	
24. Phosphorus (PO_4^-)	
25. Lactate	

26. Blood urea nitrogen (BUN) level is:
    A. directly related to protein intake.
    B. increased in gastrointestinal bleeding or diminished kidney function.
    C. decreased in liver impairment.
    D. all of the above.

27. When a person's muscle mass is stable, clearance of creatinine may be used to assess the _____ function.
    A. hepatic
    B. renal
    C. cardiac
    D. pulmonary

28. Since an elevated lactic dehydrogenase (LDH) enzyme may be caused by at least _____ different organ or system injuries, _____ should be done to identify the organ or system involved.
    A. 3; LDH differentials
    B. 3; LDH assays
    C. 5; LDH differentials
    D. 5; LDH assays

29. Cardiac enzymes are released from myocardial tissue into the serum during:
    A. low cardiac output state.
    B. myocardial injury.
    C. cardiac arrhythmia.
    D. cardiopulmonary resuscitation.

30. All of the following enzymes are useful in the assessment of myocardial injury *except:*
    A. alanine aminotransferase (ALT).
    B. serum lactate dehydrogenase (LDH).
    C. serum glutamic-oxaloacetic transaminase (SGOT).
    D. myocardial-specific creatine kinase (CKMB).

31. CKMB levels begin rising _____ hours following myocardial injury and reach a peak in _____.
    A. 4 to 8; 2 to 3 days
    B. 4 to 8; 24 hours
    C. 10 to 12; 2 to 3 days
    D. 10 to 12; 24 hours

32. The levels of amylase and lipase are elevated in:
    A. pancreatic injury.
    B. gastrointestinal abnormalities.
    C. biliary tract disease.
    D. all of the above.

33. Bilirubin is a breakdown product of _____ that is metabolized in the _____.
    A. protein; liver
    B. protein; kidney
    C. hemoglobin; liver
    D. hemoglobin; kidney

34. Serum _____ is the most common protein measured and used as a marker of _____ synthetic function and nutritional function.
    A. albumin; kidney
    B. albumin; liver
    C. glucose; kidney
    D. glucose; liver

35. Serum hyperglycemia may occur in:
    A. impairment of insulin production (type 1 diabetes).
    B. cellular resistance to insulin (type 2 diabetes).
    C. liver failure.
    D. A and B only.

Questions 36 to 38: Match the serum chemistries in Column I with the respective normal ranges in Column II. Use each answer ONCE.

Column I	Column II
36. Blood urea nitrogen (BUN)	A. <1.1 mg/dL B. 7 to 21 mg/dL C. 0.7 to 1.4 mg/dL
37. Serum creatinine	
38. Bilirubin	

39. Activated partial prothrombin time (aPTT) is a _____ test and it is useful during anticoagulation therapy using _____.
    A. coagulation; heparin
    B. coagulation; Coumadin
    C. enzyme; heparin
    D. enzyme; Coumadin

40. Hemoglobin:
    A. has a normal range of 10 to 12 g/dL for adults.
    B. level may be elevated in chronic hypoxia.
    C. level may be elevated in overhydration.
    D. plays an essential role in body immunity.

41. Clot formation is a function of _____ and the normal value ranges from _____.
    A. hemoglobins; 1.5 to $4.0 \times 10^5/mm^3$.
    B. hemoglobins; 15 to $40 \times 10^5/mm^3$.
    C. platelets; 1.5 to $4.0 \times 10^5/mm^3$.
    D. platelets; 15 to $40 \times 10^5/mm^3$.

42. Leukocytosis is:
    A. white blood count greater than $11,000/mm^3$.
    B. white blood count less than $4,000/mm^3$.
    C. platelet count greater than $11,000/mm^3$.
    D. platelet count less than $4,000/mm^3$.

43. A patient has a white blood count of $16,000/mm^3$. This may be caused by all of the following conditions *except:*
    A. infection.
    B. stress reaction.
    C. hemorrhage.
    D. diabetes.

CHAPTER 21

Arterial Blood Gases

1. Which of the following blood gas parameters is directly measured with an electrode in a blood gas analyzer?
   A. pH
   B. PCO_2
   C. PO_2
   D. All of the above

2. The site of choice for arterial puncture is the _____ artery because collateral blood flow below the puncture site is provided by the _____ artery.
   A. radial; brachial
   B. radial; ulnar
   C. ulnar; radial
   D. ulnar; brachial

3. Arrange in proper order the steps to perform Allen's test. (Note: not all steps are listed.)
   I. Observe return of blood to hand.
   II. Tighten the hand a few times to force blood from the hand.
   III. Compress radial and ulnar arteries to stop blood flow to hand.
   IV. Relax hand and release ulnar artery while keeping radial artery compressed.
   A. I, III, IV, II
   B. II, III, IV, I
   C. III, II, I, IV
   D. IV, II, I, III

4. Air-vented syringes are used for arterial blood gas collection because:
   A. arterial blood pressure is enough to fill syringe.
   B. air must be present in sample.
   C. air is used as an anticoagulant.
   D. the air-vented feature facilitates aspiration of sample.

5. After collecting the arterial blood sample, the puncture site should be compressed for at least _____ minutes or until the bleeding has stopped.
   A. one
   B. two
   C. three
   D. five

6. Common sites available for arterial blood sampling include all of the following *except*:
   A. radial artery.
   B. brachial artery.
   C. carotid artery.
   D. femoral artery.

7. During puncture of the brachial artery, the needle should not be directed towards the medial aspect of the brachial artery because puncture of the _____ is likely.
   A. median nerve
   B. somatic nerve
   C. brachial vein
   D. basilic vein

8. Capillary blood gas sample may be used:
   A. when artery sample is not available.
   B. for the assessment of pH.
   C. for the assessment of PO_2.
   D. for the assessment of PCO_2.

9. In regard to collection of capillary blood sample from the heel:
   A. the heel should be squeezed.
   B. the posterior curvature of the heel should not be punctured.
   C. punctures may be made over old puncture sites.
   D. the puncture site should be iced before sampling.

10. A significant volume of air in an arterial blood gas sample:
    A. increases the PCO_2 value.
    B. decreases the PO_2 value.
    C. increases the pH value.
    D. does not lead to meaningful errors.

11. Every eight hours, a complete calibration should be done on a blood gas analyzer. This automated procedure involves a _____-point calibration with _____ levels of control for each of the three electrodes in a blood gas analyzer.
    A. six; two
    B. four; two
    C. three; one
    D. two; one

12. The partial pressure of oxygen in the inspired gas is *least* likely to be affected by the:
    A. barometric pressure.
    B. partial pressure of water vapor.
    C. partial pressure of nitrogen.
    D. inspired oxygen concentration.

13. Based on the normal oxygen uptake pathway, the lowest level of oxygen is found in the:
    A. alveoli.
    B. inspired gas.
    C. venous blood.
    D. arterial blood.

14. Based on the characteristics of the oxyhemoglobin dissociation curve, the 90% saturation level is clinically important because:
    A. below 90% saturation, the oxygen delivery is reduced significantly.
    B. below 90% saturation, the work of breathing is reduced significantly.
    C. above 90% saturation, the oxygen consumption is reduced significantly.
    D. above 90% saturation, the PCO_2 is increased significantly.

15. The oxyhemoglobin dissociation curve is shifted to the right with:
    A. hypothermia.
    B. acidosis.
    C. hyperventilation.
    D. hypocarbia.

16. When the oxyhemoglobin dissociation curve is shifted to the left of its normal position, the:
    A. P_{50} becomes higher than 27 mm Hg.
    B. P_{50} becomes lower than 27 mm Hg.
    C. oxygen saturation at any PO_2 remains unchanged.
    D. PO_2 at any oxygen saturation remains unchanged.

17. An increased carboxyhemoglobin level causes tissue hypoxia because carbon monoxide has a much higher _____ to hemoglobin than _____.
    A. solubility coefficient; carbon dioxide
    B. solubility coefficient; oxygen
    C. affinity; carbon dioxide
    D. affinity; oxygen

18. During gas transport, carbon dioxide exists in all of the following forms *except:*
    A. dissolved carbon dioxide.
    B. hydrogen ions.
    C. carbamino compound.
    D. carbonate acid (and dissociated form).

19. Normal ventilation with a decrease in blood flow leads to a _____ V/Q ratio. This condition is known as _____.
    A. high; dead space ventilation
    B. high; shunt
    C. low; dead space ventilation
    D. low; shunt

20. Normal perfusion with a decrease in ventilation leads to a _____ V/Q ratio. This condition is known as _____.
    A. high; dead space ventilation
    B. high; shunt
    C. low; dead space ventilation
    D. low; shunt

21. Atelectasis is a condition that causes a _____ V/Q ratio or _____.
    A. high; dead space ventilation
    B. high; shunt
    C. low; dead space ventilation
    D. low; shunt

22. Gas exchange at the alveolar-capillary level is by:
    A. ventilation.
    B. perfusion.
    C. diffusion.
    D. mitochondria.

23. Mild hypoxemia in adults is defined as _____ of _____ mm Hg.
    A. PO_2; more than 80
    B. PO_2; less than 80
    C. PCO_2; more than 40
    D. PCO_2; less than 80

24. The $P(A-a)O_2$ of a 50-year-old patient is 30 mm Hg while breathing room air. This can be interpreted as:
    A. normal oxygenation status.
    B. hypoxemia.
    C. hypoventilation.
    D. hyperventilation.

25. To calculate the percent of shunting (blood flow not taking part in gas exchange), you would need all of the following measurements *except:*
    A. end-capillary oxygen content.
    B. arterial oxygen content.
    C. PO_2.
    D. mixed venous oxygen content.

26. Mr. Laws, a postoperative patient, is found to have a 5% shunt. The proper interpretation of this finding is:
    A. normal.
    B. mild shunting.
    C. moderate shunting.
    D. severe shunting.

27. Hypoxemia caused by shunting problems responds to oxygen therapy _____ because _____ is diminished in shunts.
    A. well; perfusion
    B. well; ventilation
    C. poorly; perfusion
    D. poorly; ventilation

Questions 28 to 32: Match the types of hypoxia in Column I with the respective examples in Column II. Use each answer ONCE.

Column I	Column II
28. Affinity hypoxia	A. Congestive heart failure, hypovolemia, cardiac arrest
29. Anemic hypoxia	B. Carbon monoxide poisoning, methemoglobinemia
30. Histotoxic hypoxia	C. Cyanide poisoning
	D. Lung disease, high altitude
31. Hypoxic hypoxia	E. Alkalosis
32. Stagnant hypoxia	

33. The normal mixed venous PO_2 (PvO_2) is:
    A. 20 to 25 mm Hg.
    B. 25 to 35 mm Hg.
    C. 35 to 40 mm Hg.
    D. 80 to 100 mm Hg.

34. The mixed venous PO_2 (PvO_2) for Ms. Royster is 30 mm Hg. This may be caused by:
    A. increased oxygen extraction.
    B. decreased oxygen extraction.
    C. increased ventilation.
    D. decreased ventilation.

Questions 35 to 38: Match the types of dead space in Column I with the respective descriptions in Column II. Use only FOUR answers.

Column I	Column II
35. Anatomic dead space	A. The volume in the alveoli that does not take part in gas exchange due to lack of perfusion
36. Alveolar dead space	B. The volume in the conducting airway
	C. The volume in the tubing distal to the "Y" that does not take part in gas exchange
37. Physiological dead space	D. Sum of mechanical and alveolar dead space
38. Mechanical dead space	E. Sum of anatomic and mechanical dead space
	F. Sum of anatomic and alveolar dead space

39. The acid-base balance of the blood is regulated by all of the following mechanisms *except* the:
    A. erythrocytes buffer.
    B. lungs.
    C. kidneys.
    D. electrolytes.

Questions 40 to 43: Match the types of acid-base disturbances in Column I with the examples in Column II. Use each answer ONCE.

Column I	Column II
40. Respiratory acidosis	A. Vomiting, excessive diuretic therapy
41. Respiratory alkalosis	B. Diabetes, starvation, anaerobic metabolism due to hypoxia
42. Metabolic acidosis	C. Anxiety, fever, V/Q mismatch
43. Metabolic alkalosis	D. Alveolar hypoventilation, drug overdose

Questions 44 to 47: Match the types of acid-base disturbances in Column I with the changes in pH, PCO$_2$ and HCO$_3^-$ in Column II. Use each answer ONCE.

Column I

44. Uncompensated respiratory acidosis

45. Uncompensated respiratory alkalosis

46. Uncompensated metabolic acidosis

47. Uncompensated metabolic alkalosis

Column II

A. Increased pH, decreased PCO$_2$, and normal HCO$_3^-$

B. Decreased pH, normal PCO$_2$, and decreased HCO$_3^-$

C. Decreased pH, increased PCO$_2$, and normal HCO$_3^-$

D. Increased pH, normal PCO$_2$, and increased HCO$_3^-$

48. Since an increased PCO$_2$ level in respiratory acidosis indicates _____, the primary treatment should consist of _____.
    A. hypoventilation; oxygen therapy
    B. hypoventilation; ventilation
    C. hyperventilation; oxygen therapy
    D. hyperventilation; ventilation

CHAPTER 22

Nutrition Assessment and Support

1. In short-term, the body uses glycogen and _____ as the principal fuel source for metabolic functions. In prolonged undernutrition, catabolism or breakdown of _____ (muscle tissue) occurs.
   A. fat; carbohydrate
   B. fat; protein
   C. protein; fat
   D. protein; carbohydrate

2. Catabolism of muscle tissues in prolonged starvation or undernutrition will lead to:
   A. increased metabolic rate.
   B. increased cardiac output.
   C. decreased lung functions.
   D. A and B only.

3. Depletion of phosphorus may impair oxygen release to tissues because phosphorus is an essential element in the production of:
   A. adenosine triphosphate (ATP) and 2,3-diphosphoglycerate (2,3-DPG).
   B. hemoglobin and plasma.
   C. albumin and surfactant.
   D. immunoglobulin A and neutrophils.

4. _____ deficiency may lead to muscle weakness and weaning failure from mechanical ventilation.
   A. Magnesium
   B. Phosphorus
   C. Calcium
   D. Potassium

5. Prolonged undernutrition may cause all of the following conditions *except:*
   A. depressed immune function.
   B. hyperalbuminemia.
   C. surfactant deficiency.
   D. pulmonary edema.

6. Anthropometry is the study of human:
   A. nutritional status.
   B. genetics.
   C. body functions.
   D. body measurements and components.

7. _____ is synthesized by the _____ and it is required for the transport of molecules, maintenance of the vascular system, and prevention of edema.
   A. Transferrin; liver
   B. Retino-binding protein; kidneys
   C. Albumin; liver
   D. Glycogen; bone marrow

8. With some limitations, all of the following may be used for nutritional assessment *except:*
   A. albumin and prealbumin.
   B. transferrin.
   C. retinol-binding protein.
   D. glycogen.

Questions 9 to 12: Match the biochemical measurements of nutritional status in Column I with the normal ranges in Column II. Use each answer ONCE.

Column I	Column II
9. Albumin	A. 18 to 50 mg/dL
	B. 0.0372 +/– 0.0073 g/L
10. Transferrin	C. 3.5 to 5 g/dL
	D. 200 to 400 mg/dL
11. Transthyretin (prealbumin)	
12. Retinol-binding protein	

13. Harris-Benedict equation is used to calculate a person's
_____, the amount of energy required to maintain
basic body functions.
A. energy requirement
B. cardiac index
C. basal metabolic rate
D. oxygen consumption

14. Indirect calorimetry measures the person's:
A. oxygen consumption.
B. oxygen consumption and carbon dioxide production.
C. cardiac index.
D. cardiac index and carbon dioxide production.

15. Indirect calorimetry is usually limited to patients who
are:
A. breathing spontaneously on room air.
B. mechanically ventilated with an FIO_2 less than
40%.
C. critically ill.
D. A and B only.

16. For most hospitalized patients, the measured resting
energy expenditure (REE) approximates the total
energy expenditure (TEE) because they:
A. have low metabolic rates.
B. have high metabolic rates.
C. have high energy requirements.
D. receive supplemental nutritional support.

17. For each gram of protein, it is recommended that
_____ nonprotein calories be available to the
patient.
A. 5 to 15
B. 15 to 25
C. 25 to 35
D. 35 to 45

18. Mr. King is on a diet including 80 grams of protein. If
25 nonprotein calories per gram of protein are given to
match this protein intake, how many nonprotein calo-
ries should Mr. King receive?
A. 1000 calories.
B. 1500 calories.
C. 2000 calories.
D. 2500 calories.

19. In patients without renal or liver disease, _____ of
dietary protein per kilogram of body weight should be
provided.
A. 0.6 to 1.2 g
B. 1.2 to 1.5 g
C. 1.5 to 2.0 g
D. 2.0 to 2.5 g

20. In order to prevent catabolism or an anabolic state,
the patient's _____ nitrogen balance should be
about _____ a day.
A. positive; 0 to 1 g
B. positive; 1 to 4 g
C. negative; −1 to 0 g
D. negative; −1 to −4 g

21. Enteral nutrition should be the first choice when a
patient has a functional digestive system because it:
A. promotes intestinal atrophy.
B. bypasses the intestinal tract.
C. destroys normal gut flora.
D. secretes immunoglobulins.

22. Parenteral route of nutritional support bypasses the
_____ and it is done by _____ delivery of sub-
strate.
A. gastrointestinal tract; intravenous
B. mouth; intravenous
C. blood vessels; mouth
D. blood vessels; feeding tube

23. The nutritional guidelines for patients with chronic
respiratory disease include all of the following *except:*
A. choose high-calorie, nutrient-dense foods.
B. eat small, frequent meals.
C. drink liquids between meals, not with them.
D. avoid products such as Ensure and Boost.

CHAPTER 23

Cardiac Assessment

1. The left ventricle is normally at its *fullest* level of blood volume at the _____ of _____ phase.
   A. early part; systolic
   B. early part; diastolic
   C. end; systolic
   D. end; diastolic

2. The left ventricle is normally at its *lowest* level of blood volume at the _____ of _____ phase.
   A. early part; systolic
   B. early part; diastolic
   C. end; systolic
   D. end; diastolic

3. The blood volume delivered by the left ventricle can be calculated by *subtracting* the lowest level of blood volume [_____] *from* the highest level of blood volume [_____] in the left ventricle.
   A. end-diastolic volume (EDV); end-systolic volume (ESV)
   B. end-systolic volume (ESV); end-diastolic volume (EDV)
   C. systolic volume (SV); diastolic volume (DV)
   D. diastolic volume (DV); systolic volume (SV)

4. The ejection fraction depends on all of the following factors *except*:
   A. ECG rhythms.
   B. preload conditions.
   C. heart rate.
   D. contractility.

5. Left ventricular hypertrophy may be detected by the all of the following ECG changes *except*:
   A. prolonged depolarization.
   B. repolarization abnormalities.
   C. decrease in voltage.
   D. shift in the QRS axis.

Questions 6 to 9: Match the specific tests to assess left ventricular function in Column I with the respective descriptions in Column II. Use each answer ONCE.

Column I

6. Electrocardiography

7. Radionuclide angiocardiography

8. Echocardiography

9. Cardiac catheterization

Column II

A. Pass a catheter retrograde via the femoral artery and aorta into the left ventricle and obtain the left ventriculography
B. Use ultrasonography to examine the structures and function of the left ventricle
C. Evaluate the electrical conduction of the enlarged left ventricle (i.e., shift of QRS axis)
D. Inject a radioisotope intravenously and use a special camera to detect the isotope's signal in the left ventricle

10. Diastolic dysfunction refers to an abnormality of the _____ of the left ventricle.
    A. contraction
    B. electrical conduction
    C. filling
    D. size

11. Diastolic dysfunction causes an abnormally _____ volume of blood in the _____ ventricles.
    A. high; compliant
    B. high; noncompliant
    C. low; compliant
    D. low; noncompliant

12. The standard test for evaluating left ventricular diastolic function is:
    A. echocardiography.
    B. electrocardiography.
    C. cardiac catheterization.
    D. ultrasonography.

13. Cor pulmonale is enlargement or failure of the _____ ventricle and this condition is typically related to chronic lung diseases and pulmonary _____.
    A. left; hypertension
    B. left; hypotension
    C. right; hypotension
    D. right; hypertension

14. Mr. Goldberg has an admitting diagnosis of cor pulmonale. His clinical signs may include all of the following *except:*
    A. pulmonary edema.
    B. jugular vein distension.
    C. enlargement of the liver.
    D. accumulation of fluid in the peritoneal cavity.

15. The right ventricle is highly _____ and it is very sensitive to changing afterload or _____ artery pressure.
    A. compliant; systemic
    B. compliant; pulmonary
    C. noncompliant; pulmonary
    D. noncompliant; systemic

Questions 16 to 18: Match the specific tests to assess right ventricular function in Column I with the respective descriptions in Column II. Use each answer ONCE.

Column I

16. Electrocardiography
17. Radionuclide angiocardiography
18. Echocardiography

Column II

A. Use ultrasonography to examine the structures and function of the right ventricle
B. Evaluate the electrical conduction of the enlarged right ventricle (i.e., right axis deviation)
C. Determine the ejection fraction of the right ventricle

19. Stenotic lesion of a heart valve usually involves a(n) _____ in the size of the valve orifice and _____ blood flow through it.
    A. increase; increased
    B. increase; decreased
    C. decrease; increased
    D. decrease; decreased

20. Stenotic valvular lesions result in pressure overload of the _____ heart chamber. For example, aortic stenosis causes _____ ventricular hypertrophy.
    A. upstream; left
    B. upstream; right
    C. downstream; left
    D. downstream; right

21. In stenotic valvular lesions, the heart chamber downstream from the stenosis has a _____ than the heart chamber upstream from the stenosis.
    A. higher pressure and higher blood flow
    B. higher pressure and lower blood flow
    C. lower pressure and higher blood flow
    D. lower pressure and lower blood flow

22. "Severe" valvular stenosis may be defined as a pressure gradient of more than 50 mm Hg across the _____ valve.
    A. aortic
    B. aortic or pulmonic
    C. mitral
    D. mitral or tricuspid

23. Valvular _____ is a term used to describe a portion of the ventricular volume flowing backward rather than in a normal, forward fashion.
    A. stenosis
    B. obstruction
    C. regurgitation
    D. collapse

24. With aortic regurgitation, the total blood volume ejected from the left ventricle _____ the blood volume entering the left ventricle from the pulmonary circulation.
    A. is greater than
    B. equals
    C. is less than
    D. unable to determine answer without measurements

25. Assessment of valvular function may be done by all of the following procedures *except:*
    A. echocardiography.
    B. cardiac catheterization.
    C. radionuclide angiography.
    D. cardiac stress test.

26. The pressure gradient across a stenotic valve is _____ related to the size of valve opening. In other words, a _____ pressure gradient is expected in a constricted valve.
    A. directly; high
    B. directly; low
    C. inversely; high
    D. inversely; low

27. Decrease in coronary circulation affects mainly the _____ ventricular chamber of the heart and the common patient complaint is _____.
    A. left; shortness of breath
    B. left; productive cough
    C. right; shortness of breath
    D. right; productive cough

28. Based on the "ischemic cascade of cardiac dysfunction" in the text, _____ and myocardial infarction are the results of prolonged coronary ischemia.
    A. diastolic dysfunction
    B. systolic dysfunction
    C. ECG changes
    D. angina

29. List the following events in proper order from the onset of ischemia to the development of myocardial infarction.
    I. ECG abnormalities
    II. Systolic dysfunction
    III. Diastolic dysfunction
    IV. Angina
    A. Ischemia, I, III, II, IV, myocardial infarction
    B. Ischemia, II, I, IV, III, myocardial infarction
    C. Ischemia, III, II, I, IV, myocardial infarction
    D. Ischemia, IV, II, III, I, myocardial infarction

Questions 30 to 33: Match the cardiac abnormalities in Column I with the respective ECG characteristics in Column II. You may use any answer MORE THAN ONCE.

Column I	Column II
30. Ischemia	A. Displacement of ST segment
	B. Q wave change
31. Myocardial injury	C. T wave change
32. Recent myocardial infarction	
33. Old myocardial infarction	

34. In Figure B above, the arrows in leads V_4 to V_6 show:
    A. ST segment depression.
    B. P wave change.
    C. inverted Q wave.
    D. upright U wave.

35. The ECG change from the previous question is caused by:
    A. valvular stenosis.
    B. congenital heart defect.
    C. myocardial infarction.
    D. myocardial ischemia.

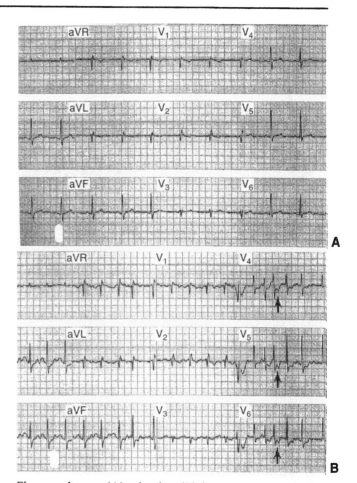

Electrocardiogram (A) at baseline (B) during exercise treadmill test at peak heart rate.

36. Exercise stress testing is one of the available tests to assess coronary circulation because exercise _____ the myocardial _____.
    A. increases; oxygen demand
    B. increases; compliance
    C. decreases; oxygen demand
    D. decreases; compliance

37. For patients who are unable to exercise, coronary circulation may be assessed by using dobutamine because it has the ability to increase a patient's:
    A. heart rate.
    B. systolic blood pressure.
    C. myocardial contractility.
    D. all of the above.

38. Coronary arteriography performed during cardiac catheterization is the standard test for the assessment of:
    A. electrical conductivity of the heart.
    B. coronary circulation.
    C. cardiac output.
    D. myocardial contractility.

CHAPTER 24

Imaging the Thorax

1. Chest radiography is typically done by projecting x-rays through the chest _____ and the air-filled structures appear _____ on the radiography.
   A. from anterior to posterior; black
   B. from anterior to posterior; white
   C. from posterior to anterior; black
   D. from posterior to anterior; white

2. The bony structures appear _____ on the radiography because they have high density and are able to absorb _____ of the x-ray energy.
   A. white; most
   B. white; little
   C. black; most
   D. black; little

3. A posterior-anterior (PA) projection of the chest is preferred over an anterior-posterior (AP) projection because:
   A. the heart size is not magnified with a PA projection.
   B. a PA projection is easier to perform in a critical care unit.
   C. the cost for a PA projection is less.
   D. all of the above.

4. In order to evaluate the lung bases and lung parenchyma behind the heart, a(n) _____ chest radiography is recommended.
   A. lordotic
   B. expiratory
   C. lateral
   D. oblique

5. Referring to the figure shown on page 69, _____ represents the location of the aortic knob.
   A. 1
   B. 4
   C. 8
   D. 9

6. Abnormalities within the lung or pleura that produce radiodense processes are called:
   A. radiodensities.
   B. opacities.
   C. air bronchograms.
   D. silhouette signs.

7. _____ occurs when an opacified area of the lung causes the border between two structures to become obliterated.
   A. Air bronchogram
   B. Silhouette sign
   C. Contrast
   D. Radiopaque

8. Air bronchogram occurs when the _____ bronchi are present with _____ lung parenchyma.
   A. fluid-filled; air-filled
   B. fluid-filled; fluid-filled
   C. air-filled; air-filled
   D. air-filled; fluid-filled

9. On the chest radiography, one feature that distinguishes between atelectasis and pneumonia is that:
   A. pneumonia produces bilateral abnormalities.
   B. atelectasis produces bilateral abnormalities.
   C. pneumonia may appear and disappear rapidly.
   D. atelectasis may appear and disappear rapidly.

10. Radiographic signs of atelectasis may include all of the following *except*:
    A. displacement of fissures toward the unaffected side.
    B. increased radiopacity.
    C. air bronchogram.
    D. hemidiaphragm elevation on the affected side.

11. Radiographic signs of pneumonia may include all of the following *except:*
    A. air bronchogram.
    B. hemidiaphragms are not elevated.
    C. lung volume is reduced.
    D. increased radiopacity.

12. In cardiogenic pulmonary edema, the radiographic signs may include all of the following *except:*
    A. visible edema in connecting tissue around the vessels and airways.
    B. enlarged heart.
    C. gravitationally distributed edema.
    D. initial involvement in the upper lobes.

13. The best radiographic study for pulmonary embolism is:
    A. pulmonary angiography.
    B. chest radiography.
    C. ventilation/perfusion scan.
    D. computed tomography.

14. _____ is the standard test for diagnosis of deep vein thrombosis in the lower extremities.
    A. Magnetic resonance imaging (MRI)
    B. Contrast venography
    C. Duplex ultrasound
    D. Angiography

15. As a diagnostic tool, MRI is:
    A. inexpensive.
    B. popular because of ease of patient monitoring.
    C. limited because routine radiography provides similar information.
    D. not suitable for patients with a cardiac pacemaker.

16. Expiratory chest radiography enhances the visualization of the _____ pleura. This technique is used to rule out _____.
    A. parietal; pneumothorax
    B. visceral; pneumothorax
    C. parietal; pneumomediastinum
    D. visceral; pneumothorax

17. In reviewing a patient's chest radiography, you notice that the tip of an endotracheal tube is about 2 cm from the carina. You would _____ the tube until the tip is about _____ from the carina.
    A. advance; 0.5 cm
    B. advance; 1 cm
    C. withdraw; 4 cm
    D. withdraw; 4 in

18. A properly placed central venous catheter should have the distal tip:
    A. at the junction of the brachiocephalic vein and superior vena cava.
    B. at the junction of the cephalic vein and inferior vena cava.
    C. proximal to the left atrium.
    D. proximal to the inferior vena cava.

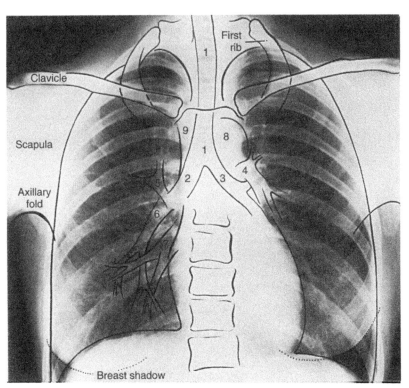

Posterior projection of normal chest film.

Questions 19 to 22: Match the imagine techniques in Column I with the respective characteristics in Column II. Use each answer ONCE.

Column I

19. Radiography (x-ray)

20. Computed tomography (CT)

21. Magnetic resonance imaging (MRI)

22. Positron enhanced tomography (PET)

Column II

A. Contraindicated in patients with cardiac pacemaker

B. Provides physiologic and metabolic information, ideal for evaluation of tumors

C. Exposes patient to ionizing radiation

D. Inexpensive and most common radiographic study

CHAPTER 25

Pulmonary Function Testing

1. Restrictive lung diseases show _____ in a pulmonary function study, whereas obstructive lung diseases show _____.
    A. increased flow rates; decreased flow rates
    B. increased volumes; decreased volumes
    C. decreased flow rates; increased flow rates
    D. decreased volumes; decreased flow rates

2. The lungs are divided into _____ lung volumes and _____ lung capacities.
    A. three; five
    B. four; four
    C. four; five
    D. five, three

Questions 3 to 6: Match the lung volumes in Column I with the descriptions in Column II. Use each answer ONCE.

Column I

3. Tidal volume (V_T)

4. Inspiratory reserve volume (IRV)

5. Expiratory reserve volume (ERV)

6. Residual volume (RV)

Column II

A. Maximum volume of gas that can be *expired* from the end of a normal tidal expiration.

B. Volume of gas that remains in the lungs after a maximal expiration.

C. Maximum volume of gas that can be *inspired* from the end of a normal tidal inspiration.

D. Volume of gas inhaled or exhaled during normal breathing.

7. There are _____ lung capacities and each lung capacity contains at least _____ lung volumes.
    A. three; two
    B. three; three
    C. four; two
    D. four; three

Questions 8 to 11: Match the lung capacities in Column I with the descriptions in Column II. Use each answer ONCE.

Column I

8. Vital capacity (VC)

9. Inspiratory capacity (IC)

10. Functional residual capacity (FRC)

11. Total lung capacity (TLC)

Column II

A. Maximum volume of gas that can be inspired from the end-tidal expiration level (sum of IRV and V_T).

B. Volume of gas in the lungs after a maximal inspiration (sum of IRV, V_T, ERV, and RV).

C. Maximum volume of gas that can be expired from the lungs after a maximal inspiration (sum of IRV, V_T, and ERV).

D. Volume of gas remaining in the lungs at the end-tidal expiration level (sum of ERV and RV).

12. In pulmonary function testing, _____ can be measured directly.
    A. vital capacity
    B. residual volume
    C. functional residual capacity
    D. total lung capacity

13. For lung volume/capacities that cannot be measured directly, all of the following indirect methods may be used *except*:
    A. nitrogen washout.
    B. diffusion study.
    C. helium dilution.
    D. body plethysmography.

14. Mr. Pendleton, a patient with COPD, is ready for an initial pulmonary function study. Since the physician wants to evaluate the gas volume trapped behind obstructions, you would use _____ to complete this study.
    A. body plethysmography
    B. helium dilution and nitrogen washout
    C. nitrogen washout and radiographic estimation
    D. helium dilution and body plethysmography

15. Normal predicted values are usually based on a person's:
    A. age.
    B. gender.
    C. height.
    D. all of the above.

16. Pulmonary function testing on Ms. Jones has the following selected results: VC = 81% predicted, FRC = 118% predicted. These two measurements:
    A. are within normal range.
    B. reveal technical errors.
    C. show that VC is too low and FRC is too high.
    D. show that VC and FRC are both too high.

17. Mr. Caine has a history of COPD and air trapping. You would expect to see all of the following measurements to be elevated *except:*
    A. RV.
    B. FRC.
    C. V_T.
    D. TLC.

18. Hyperinflation of the lung parenchyma can be documented by an elevated:
    A. RV.
    B. FRC.
    C. RV/TLC.
    D. TLC.

19. Reduced lung volumes and capacities are indicative of:
    A. obstructive disease.
    B. restrictive disease.
    C. diffusion defects.
    D. perfusion defects.

20. Elevated residual volume or total lung capacity is a sign of _____ and is indicative of _____.
    A. air trapping or hyperinflation; obstructive disease
    B. air trapping or hyperinflation; restrictive disease
    C. air trapping; diffusion defects
    D. hyperinflation; perfusion defects

21. The lung volume recorded in one second during a forced vital capacity maneuver is called _____ and this is used to evaluate presence and severity of _____.
    A. FEF_1; small airway obstruction
    B. FEV_1; large airway obstruction
    C. FEF_1/FVC; small airway obstruction
    D. FEV_1/FVC; large airway obstruction

22. The flow rate measured during the middle half of a forced vital capacity maneuver is called _____ and this is used to evaluate presence and severity of _____.
    A. FEF_{50}; small airway obstruction
    B. FEV_{50}; large airway obstruction
    C. $FEF_{25-75\%}$; small airway obstruction
    D. $FEV_{25-75\%}$; large airway obstruction

23. Pulmonary function testing on Ms. Warren has the following selected results: FEV_1 = 54% predicted, FEV_1/FVC = 87%. These two measurements indicate that she may have:
    A. small airway obstruction.
    B. large airway obstruction.
    C. restrictive lung disease.
    D. restrictive and obstructive lung disease.

24. Mr. Arnold has completed a pulmonary function test and two of the measurements are: FEV_1 = 62% predicted; FEV_1/FVC = 60%. These two measurements indicate that he may have:
    A. small airway obstruction.
    B. large airway obstruction.
    C. restrictive lung disease.
    D. restrictive and obstructive lung disease.

25. Ms. Queen, an outpatient in the pulmonary function laboratory, has finished a pre- and postbronchodilator study. The results show: prebronchodilator FEV_1 = 1.0 L and postbronchodilator FEV_1 = 1.2 L. This represents _____ improvement and it is considered _____.
    A. 2%; significant and reversible obstruction
    B. 2%; insignificant and irreversible obstruction
    C. 20%; significant and reversible obstruction
    D. 20%; insignificant and irreversible obstruction

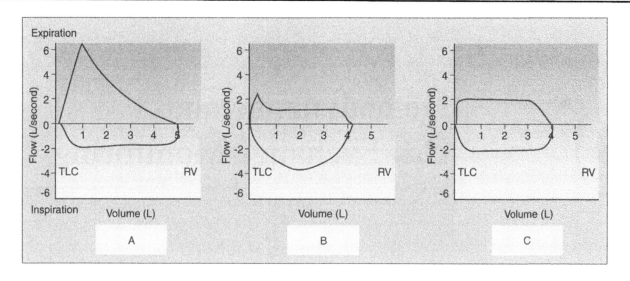

26. In the figure provided above, illustration "A" shows a typical flow-volume loop from a person with _____ lesion and the FEF_{50}/FIF_{50} is _____ than 1.
    A. intrathoracic; greater
    B. intrathoracic; less
    C. extrathoracic; greater
    D. extrathoracic; less

27. FEV_6 may be used to replace FVC as a(n) _____ criterion and it helps to avoid _____ in office spirometry.
    A. obstructive; exertion
    B. restrictive; hypoxia
    C. obstructive and restrictive; exertion and hypoxia
    D. end of test; exertion

28. Carbon monoxide (CO) is an ideal gas for _____ study because of its _____.
    A. peak flow; high density
    B. peak flow; low density
    C. diffusion; high diffusion coefficient
    D. diffusion; low diffusion coefficient

29. In bronchial challenge testing, methacholine or histamine is used to induce:
    A. bronchoconstriction.
    B. bronchodilation.
    C. vasoconstriction.
    D. vasodilation.

30. Referring to the figure shown below, the onset of airway closure during a single breath nitrogen washout study is represented by phase _____.
    A. I
    B. II
    C. III
    D. IV

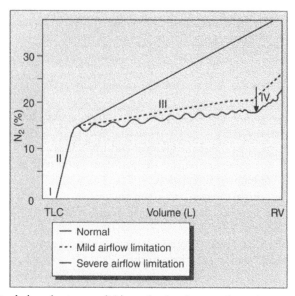

Single-breath nitrogen (N_2) test for distribution of ventilation with normal lung function, mild obstructive lung disease, and significant maldistribution of ventilation.

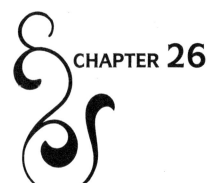

CHAPTER 26

Hemodynamic and Gas Exchange Monitoring

1. Telemetry and Holter monitors are used to monitor _____ and they are typically used _____ the intensive care unit.
   A. heart rate; in
   B. heart rate; outside
   C. heart rate and rhythm; in
   D. heart rate and rhythm; outside

2. You are asked to place an arterial catheter on a critically ill patient. Your first choice of site placement would be the _____ artery.
   A. ulnar
   B. femoral
   C. brachial
   D. radial

3. In regard to the use and care of a central venous catheter, the:
   A. reading should be taken at end-inspiration.
   B. measurement reflects the perfusion status of the pulmonary circulation.
   C. normal range is 0 to 7 mm Hg.
   D. proper position is in the pulmonary vein.

4. The CVP readings for Mr. Jones have been between 4 and 6 mm Hg over the past three days. On your most recent ICU rounds, you notice that his CVP reading stays around 2 mm Hg. You would assess the patient for signs of:
   A. hypervolemia.
   B. hypovolemia.
   C. hyperventilation.
   D. hypoventilation.

5. Dr. Howe asks you to assist her in placing a catheter for the monitoring of cardiac output, right ventricular ejection fraction, and mixed venous oxygen content. You would assume that Dr. Howe is putting in a(n):
   A. pulmonary artery catheter.
   B. arterial catheter.
   C. central venous catheter.
   D. suction catheter.

Questions 6 to 10: Match the hemodynamic measurements in Column I with the normal ranges in Column II. Use each answer ONCE.

Column I

6. Systolic blood pressure

7. Right atrial (central venous) pressure

8. Pulmonary artery systolic pressure

9. Pulmonary artery diastolic pressure

10. Pulmonary artery wedge pressure

Column II

A. 2 to 12 mm Hg
B. 4 to 12 mm Hg
C. 0 to 8 mm Hg
D. 100 to 140 mm Hg
E. 15 to 30 mm Hg

11. As you are making rounds in the CCU, you notice that the pressure transducer for Mr. Rite's pulmonary artery catheter is several inches below his midaxillary line. This condition would:
    A. not affect the actual pressure readings.
    B. lead to higher-than-actual pressure readings.
    C. lead to lower-than-actual pressure readings.
    D. cause backup of blood into the catheter.

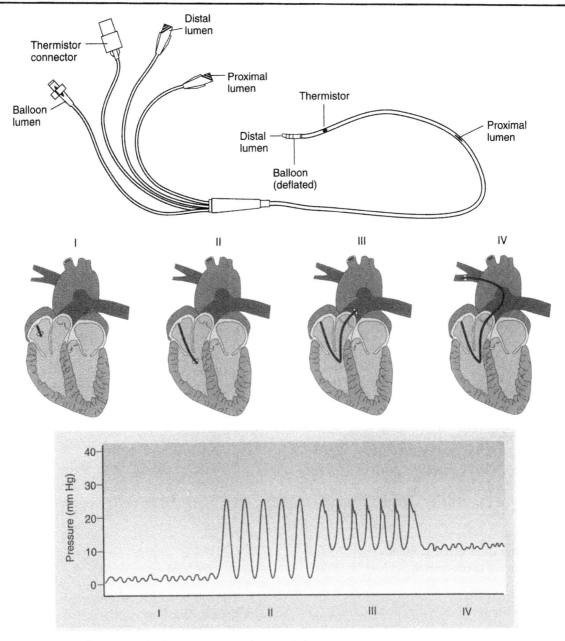

Conventional pulmonary artery catheter and characteristic pressure waveforms.

12. From the pressure waveforms shown in figure above, the second set of waveform (II) occurs when the distal end of a pulmonary artery catheter is in the:
    A. right atrium.
    B. right ventricle.
    C. pulmonary artery.
    D. left ventricle.

13. Based on the Fick equation, cardiac output has _____ relationship with the oxygen consumption rate when the arterial mixed-venous oxygen content difference is held constant.
    A. a direct
    B. an inverse
    C. a variable
    D. no

14. During exercise testing, the most accurate indirect method to monitor tidal volume changes is the:
    A. impedance pneumography.
    B. piezoelectric plethysmography.
    C. fiberoptic plethysmography.
    D. respiratory inductance plethysmography.

15. In comparison to traditional larger blood gas analyzers, point of care analyzers have all of the following advantages *except*:
    A. quicker turnaround time.
    B. lower overhead cost.
    C. smaller sample size required.
    D. more testing capability.

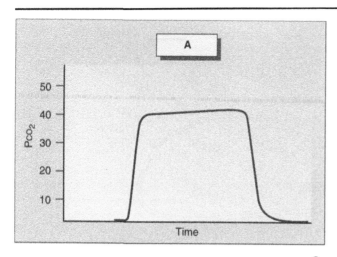

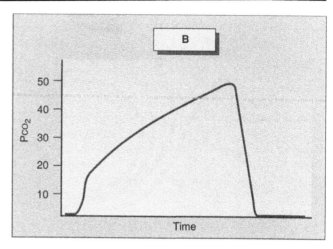

Capnograms.

16. Since transcutaneous PO_2 monitoring requires _____ perfusion to the skin surface, a low $P_{TC}O_2/PaO_2$ ratio reflects _____.
    A. sufficient; high cardiac index
    B. sufficient; low cardiac index
    C. minimal; high cardiac index
    D. minimal; low cardiac index

Questions 17 to 21. Ms. Rule, a patient who is breathing spontaneously in the emergency department, has the following blood gas results: pH = 7.44, $PaCO_2$= 34 mm Hg, PaO_2 = 100 mm Hg, SaO_2 = 77%, COHb = 18%, F_IO_2= 21%. The patient's SpO_2 at the time of arterial puncture was 99%.

17. With the information given above, the _____ measurement is out of normal range.
    A. pH
    B. $PaCO_2$
    C. PaO_2
    D. SaO_2

18. With the information given above, the _____ measurement does not correlate with the rest of the results.
    A. $PaCO_2$
    B. SaO_2
    C. SpO_2
    D. CaO_2

19. With the information given above, the discrepancy or error is between:
    A. $PaCO_2$ and PaO_2.
    B. SpO_2 and SaO_2.
    C. SpO_2 and CaO_2.
    D. SaO_2 and CaO_2.

20. With the information given above, the lack of correlation with one measurement is because this measurement tends to:
    A. become inaccurate when the F_IO_2 is less than 40%.
    B. become inaccurate when no supplemental oxygen is provided.
    C. overestimate the value in the presence of abnormal hemoglobin.
    D. underestimate the value in the presence of abnormal hemoglobin.

21. With the information given above, you would alert the physician that the _____ is the cause of the problem and the patient should be treated accordingly.
    A. COHb
    B. SpO_2
    C. PaO_2
    D. SaO_2

22. The end-tidal CO_2 represents the _____ and the normal value is near _____.
    A. arterial pCO_2; 40 mm Hg
    B. arterial pCO_2; 100 mm Hg
    C. alveolar pCO_2; 40 mm Hg
    D. alveolar pCO_2; 100 mm Hg

23. Referring to the illustrations above, Figure A represents the capnogram in healthy subjects and Figure B represents the capnogram in patients with:
    A. COPD.
    B. restrictive lung disease.
    C. small airway obstruction.
    D. obstructive and restrictive lung disease.

24. When applied appropriately to the patient condition, capnogram may be used in all of the following clinical situations *except*:
    A. assessment of intrapulmonary shunting.
    B. detection of dead space ventilation.
    C. assessment of endotracheal intubation.
    D. evaluation of CPR effectiveness.

Questions 25 to 27. Mr. Samford, a patient with congestive heart failure, has the following blood gas results: Arterial pH = 7.38, $PaCO_2$ = 43 mm Hg, PaO_2 = 100 mm Hg, SaO_2 = 98%. Mixed venous pH = 7.34, $PvCO_2$ = 49 mm Hg, PvO_2 = 60 mm Hg, SvO_2 = 78%, F_IO_2 = 21%. Hemoglobin = 15 g/dL.

25. With the information given above, the *arterial* oxygen content (CaO_2) is about:
    A. 16 vol%.
    B. 18 vol%.
    C. 20 vol%.
    D. 22 vol%.

26. With the information given above, the *mixed venous* oxygen content (CvO_2) is about:
    A. 16 vol%.
    B. 18 vol%.
    C. 20 vol%.
    D. 22 vol%.

27. With the information given above, the oxygen extraction ratio (O_2ER) is about:
    A. 10%.
    B. 20%.
    C. 30%.
    D. 40%.

Questions 28 to 30. Ms. Tomlin, a patient with COPD, has the following measurements: cardiac output = 6 L/min, heart rate = 100/min, body surface area = 1.2 m^2.

28. With the information given above, the stroke volume is:
    A. 20 mL/beat.
    B. 40 mL/beat.
    C. 60 mL/beat.
    D. 72 mL/beat.

29. With the information given above, the cardiac index is:
    A. 1.6 L/min/m^2.
    B. 5 L/min/m^2.
    C. 7.2 L/min/m^2.
    D. 15 L/min/m^2.

30. With the information given above, the stroke volume index is:
    A. 30 mL/beat/m^2.
    B. 40 mL/beat/m^2.
    C. 50 mL/beat/m^2.
    D. 60 mL/beat/m^2.

31. Since _____ correlates well with serum lactate and tissue acidosis, it may be used as an endpoint for resuscitation.
    A. base deficit
    B. base excess
    C. mixed venous oxygen saturation
    D. arterial oxygen saturation

32. Monitoring equipment in a critical care environment is typically composed of:
    A. sensors and transducers.
    B. signal transmission components.
    C. signal processing components.
    D. all of the above.

CHAPTER **27**

Exercise Assessment

Questions 1 to 3: You are observing an exercise testing on an outpatient in the cardiopulmonary stress laboratory. Mr. Lamb is 40 years old and has a diagnosis of dyspnea on exertion.

1. The advantage of exercise testing is that the results are _____ measurements and they may be used to evaluate a patient's _____.
   A. dynamic; functional status
   B. dynamic; best efforts
   C. static; functional status
   D. static; best efforts

2. During the initial stage of testing, you would expect to Mr. Lamb to have an increasing:
   A. oxygen consumption.
   B. heart rate.
   C. respiratory rate.
   D. all of the above.

3. To measure Mr. Lamb's oxygen consumption, all of the following parameters must be known *except:*
   A. CaO_2.
   B. CvO_2.
   C. CcO_2.
   D. cardiac output.

4. Based on the equation VO_2 = cardiac output $\times$ (CaO_2–CvO_2), (CaO_2–CvO_2) represents:
   A. oxygen extraction rate.
   B. oxygen delivery rate.
   C. oxygen content.
   D. stroke volume.

5. Mr. Thomas, an outpatient with no known cardiopulmonary abnormalities, is getting ready to use the treadmill. At the early stage of the test, you would anticipate all of the following physiologic responses *except:*
   A. increase in minute ventilation.
   B. decrease in blood pressure.
   C. increase in cardiac output.
   D. decrease in systemic vascular resistance.

6. If the oxygen consumption (VO_2) and carbon dioxide production (VCO_2) of a patient are 3.0 L and 2.5 L, respectively, the calculated respiratory exchange ratio is about:
   A. 0.6.
   B. 0.8.
   C. 1.2.
   D. 1.4.

7. Before exercise testing, a patient's resting minute ventilation is 6 L/min. As testing progresses, you would expect to see an increase in:
   A. minute ventilation.
   B. respiratory rate.
   C. tidal volume.
   D. all of the above.

8. Since a higher-than-normal _____ is a common characteristic in COPD patients, the end-expiratory lung volume for these patients during exercise impinges on the _____.
   A. vital capacity; residual volume
   B. vital capacity; tidal volume
   C. functional residual capacity; inspiratory capacity
   D. functional residual capacity; expiratory reserve volume

9. Since the anatomic dead space is _____ during exercise, shallow breathing leads to a(n) _____ dead space to tidal volume (V_D/V_T) ratio.
   A. increased; increased
   B. decreased; decreased
   C. unchanged; increased
   D. variable; decreased

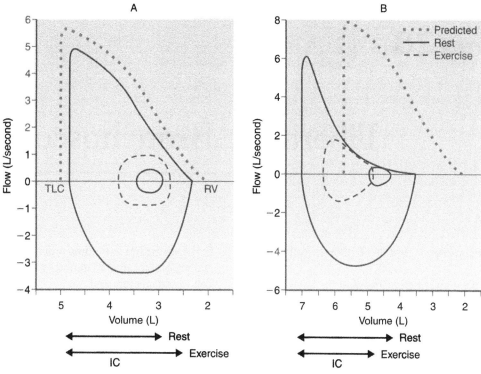

Flow volume loops.

10. Referring to the above illustrations, Figure A represents the flow volume loops in healthy subjects and Figure B represents the flow volume loops in patients with:
   A. COPD.
   B. restrictive lung disease.
   C. small airway obstruction.
   D. obstructive and restrictive lung disease.

11. The following pCO_2 measurements are obtained from a patient during exercise testing, what is the calculated dead space to tidal volume (V_D/V_T) ratio?

   $PaCO_2 = 40$ mm Hg, $P_ECO_2 = 30$ mm Hg

   A. 10%
   B. 25%
   C. 33%
   D. 75%

12. If the base excess drops to −1 or lower during exercise, it indicates that the patient has reached the:
   A. lactate threshold.
   B. maximum cardiac output.
   C. oxygen pulse.
   D. ventilatory equivalent.

13. Fick equation is used to calculate a patient's:
   A. cardiac output.
   B. oxygen consumption.
   C. carbon dioxide production.
   D. oxygen pulse.

14. Based on the six-minute walk test, the patient may:
   A. not use bronchodilator before the test.
   B. not use supplemental oxygen during the test
   C. rest during the test as needed during the six-minute period.
   D. talk during the test.

15. Indications for cardiopulmonary exercise testing include all of the following *except*:
   A. assessment of intervention and prognosis.
   B. unexplained or disproportionate shortness of breath.
   C. pretest for pulmonary rehabilitation program.
   D. treatment of exercise-induced asthma.

16. An abnormal cardiovascular response during exercise testing includes:
   A. high lactate threshold.
   B. decreased oxygen pulse.
   C. decreased heart rate-versus-work rate relationship.
   D. all of the above.

17. Exercise testing should be terminated immediately when the:
   A. SpO_2 is less than 85%.
   B. ECG shows heart rate of 120/min.
   C. systolic blood pressure is greater than 200 mm Hg.
   D. patient complaints of lightheadedness.

CHAPTER 28

Fiberoptic Bronchoscopy

1. Fiberoptic bronchoscopy is capable of all of the following *except:*
   A. measuring pulmonary hemodynamics.
   B. viewing the inside of conducting airway.
   C. placing a stent.
   D. collecting laboratory samples.

2. The absolute contraindications for fiberoptic bronchoscopy is:
   A. hypercarbia at rest.
   B. ischemic heart disease.
   C. uncontrolled hypoxemia.
   D. cardiac arrhythmia.

Questions 3 to 6: Match the steps in preparing a patient for bronchoscopy in Column I with the rationales in Column II. Use each answer ONCE.

Column I

3. Use of lidocaine

4. Provide intravenous sedation

5. Mandatory 8-hour fasting

6. Use of atropine

Column II

A. To inhibit secretions
B. To minimize aspiration
C. To alleviate anxiety
D. To suppress coughing during procedure

Questions 7 to 8. Dr. Manning asks you to assist in a flexible bronchoscopy procedure on Ms. Jones, a patient with persistent pneumonia.

7. Prior to the procedure, you would make sure that all of the following monitoring equipment and supplies are ready *except:*
   A. arterial line access.
   B. continuous ECG monitoring.
   C. continuous pulse oximeter.
   D. intravenous (IV) access.

8. Dr. Manning has a standing order for bronchoscopy of 300 mg of lidocaine 20 minutes prior to the procedure. You would measure and use _____ mL of 4% lidocaine solution. (Given: 1 mL of a 4% lidocaine solution contains 40 mg of active ingredient.)
   A. 4
   B. 7.5
   C. 12
   D. 16

9. Many anatomical structures may be evaluated during an airway exam with a flexible bronchoscope. Select the list of anatomical structures below in their proper sequence, starting from the uppermost structure.
   I. Trachea
   II. Epiglottis
   III. Vocal cords
   IV. Posterior nasopharynx and larynx
   A. II, IV, III, and I
   B. II, III, I, and IV
   C. IV, II, III, and I
   D. IV, III, II, and I

10. During flexible bronchoscopy, orientation to the location of the bronchoscope and bronchial division is maintained by reference to the:
    A. carina.
    B. left main stem bronchus.
    C. epiglottis.
    D. trachea.

11. During bronchoalveolar lavage, up to _____ mL of _____ may be used.
    A. 100; sterile water
    B. 300; sterile water
    C. 100; saline
    D. 300; saline

12. With bronchoscopic brushing, a catheter with a brush at its distal end is introduced through the _____ channel and the brush is used to dislodge _____ along the proximal airways.
    A. irrigation; cells and tissues
    B. irrigation; mucus and blood
    C. working; cells and tissues
    D. working; mucus and blood

13. The advantage of using a protected brush during bronchoscopic brushing is that the:
    A. physician and assistant are protected from spills.
    B. sample is protected from contamination.
    C. patient is protected from excessive airway irritation.
    D. physician and assistant are protected from the patient's coughs.

14. Since endobronchial biopsy uses a _____, the major complication is _____.
    A. forceps; pneumothorax
    B. forceps; bleeding
    C. needle; pneumothorax
    D. needle; bleeding

15. With transbronchial needle aspiration, the needle is shielded inside a plastic catheter within the bronchoscope. For this reason, the needle:
    A. must be tested by exposing it while within the bronchoscope.
    B. must not be exposed while within the bronchoscope.
    C. may be reused without changing up to 20 times.
    D. may be reused after proper sterilization.

16. During transbronchial biopsy, fluoroscopy is used to provide all of the following *except:*
    A. guide the advancement of forceps.
    B. obtain sufficient sample.
    C. obtain sedation.
    D. minimize incidence of pneumothorax.

17. Since rigid bronchoscopy is less comfortable than flexible bronchoscopy, the procedure often requires:
    A. general anesthesia.
    B. neuromuscular blockade.
    C. heavy sedation.
    D. all of the above.

18. Potential complications of rigid bronchoscopy include all of the following *except:*
    A. damage to the sinus.
    B. damage to the teeth.
    C. damage to the lower respiratory tract mucosa.
    D. spasm of the larynx or bronchi.

Questions 19 to 24: Match the techniques or procedures in bronchoscopy in Column I with the applications in Column II. Use each answer ONCE.

Column I

19. Bronchoalveolar lavage
20. Bronchoscopic washing
21. Bronchoscopic brushing
22. Endobronchial biopsy
23. Transbronchial biopsy
24. Transbronchial needle aspiration

Column II

A. To diagnose submucosal infiltrates or extrinsic compressing tumors; to assist in preoperative staging of tumor
B. To sample the cellular and microbiologic components of the alveolar space
C. To sample visible central tumors or mucus ulceration
D. To sample the cellular and microbiologic components of the airway
E. To obtain cytologic samples from the proximal airways or tumors
F. To sample peripheral parenchymal masses and diagnose interstitial lung diseases

25. In terms of diagnostics, indications for bronchoscopy may include:
    A. suspected tumor or infectious disease.
    B. suspected foreign body aspiration.
    C. interstitial lung disease.
    D. all of the above.

26. Therapeutic indications for bronchoscopy include:
    A. difficult intubations.
    B. endobronchial placement of encapsulated radionuclide near tumor.
    C. stent placement to relieve obstruction.
    D. all of the above.

CHAPTER 29

Sleep Assessment

1. In nonrapid eye movement (non-REM) sleep, stages 1 and 2 are considered _____, whereas stages 3 and 4 are called deep sleep or _____ sleep.
   A. wakefulness; slow wave
   B. wakefulness; fast-wave
   C. light sleep; slow wave
   D. light sleep; fast-wave

2. In rapid eye movement (REM) sleep, the electroencephalographic (EEG) pattern is similar to that of _____ and the muscle tone is _____.
   A. wakefulness; reduced
   B. wakefulness; increased
   C. deep sleep; reduced
   D. deep sleep; increased

3. A normal sleep cycle begins with _____ and ends with _____.
   A. stage 1; stage 4
   B. stage 2; REM sleep
   C. awakened state; stage 4
   D. awakened state; REM sleep

4. During sleep, a person's _____ is increased due to _____.
   A. pCO_2; chemoreceptor responses
   B. metabolic rate; REM sleep
   C. airway resistance; changes in the muscle tone
   D. pO_2; changes in sleep cycles

5. Due to changes in a person's tonic and phasic activities during sleep, the tidal volume is primarily supported by the:
   A. intercostal muscles.
   B. accessory muscles.
   C. diaphragm.
   D. A and B only.

6. Airflow obstruction during sleep may be caused by:
   A. decreased activity of the genioglossus muscle.
   B. decreased activity of the palatal muscle group.
   C. increased activity of the infrahyoid muscle group.
   D. A and B only.

7. Mr. Lawson, a patient with COPD, has diminished respiratory drive and increased airflow resistance during sleep. You would expect _____ in his blood gas report.
   A. hypercapnia
   B. hypoxemia
   C. respiratory alkalosis
   D. A and B only

Questions 8 to 13: Match the monitoring techniques in sleep assessment in Column I with the respective descriptions in Column II. Use each answer ONCE.

Column I

8. Overnight polysomnogram

9. CPAP titration

10. Electrooculography (EOG)

11. Electromyography (EMG)

12. Oxygen plethysmograph

13. Electroencephalography (EEG)

Column II

A. To find the best airway pressure level for the patient
B. To record the brain activities during sleep
C. To monitor different neurological, cardiac, and respiratory parameters
D. To monitor and document the pulse oximetry saturation level over a period of time
E. To record the tonic and phasic muscle activity
F. To record the eye movement during sleep

14. During a sleep study, you notice that the patient's airflow has diminished despite of persistent respiratory effort. This is a sign of _____ apnea.
    A. central
    B. obstructive
    C. sleep
    D. mixed

15. Airflow may be monitored by:
    A. CO_2 detectors.
    B. thermistors or thermocouplers.
    C. pneumotachography.
    D. all of the above.

16. Strain gauges, esophageal pressure monitor, impedance pneumography, and inductive plethysmography are devices used in the measurement of:
    A. air flow.
    B. ventilatory effort.
    C. sleep stages.
    D. airway resistance.

17. In reviewing a patient's sleep study report, the calculated apnea/hypopnea index is 4 per hour. You would interpret this result as:
    A. normal.
    B. mild sleep apnea.
    C. moderate sleep apnea.
    D. severe sleep apnea.

18. The arousal index is calculated by dividing the number of arousals by the:
    A. length of each arousal.
    B. length of sleep time.
    C. number of hypopnea episodes.
    D. number of apnea episodes.

19. Apnea/hypopnea index and arousal index may be influenced by a person's _____ during a sleep study. For this reason, this observation should be noted in the report.
    A. position
    B. eye movement
    C. leg movement
    D. oxygen saturation

CHAPTER 30

Infant Apnea Monitoring

1. Based on current medical information, sudden infant death syndrome (SIDS):
   A. can be predicted in some cases.
   B. can be prevented in some cases.
   C. is caused by secondhand smoke.
   D. is linked to heredity.

2. Apnea of prematurity occurs in about _____ of preterm births and the incidence is related to the infant's _____.
   A. 25%; gestational age
   B. 25%; gestational age and birth weight
   C. 50%; birth weight
   D. 50%; gestational age and birth weight

Questions 3 to 7: Match the terms related to apnea in Column I with the respective definitions in Column II. Use each answer ONCE.

Column I

3. Pathologic apnea
4. Periodic breathing
5. Apnea of prematurity (AOP)
6. Apparent life-threatening event (ALTE)
7. Apnea of infancy

Column II

A. Periodic breathing with pathologic apnea in a premature infant usually ends by 37-weeks gestational age.
B. An unexplained episode of cessation of breathing lasting more than 20 seconds or a shorter respiratory pause associated with bradycardia, cyanosis, pallor or hypotonia. Generally refers to infants older than 37-weeks gestational age.
C. An episode that is characterized by apnea, change in color and muscle tone, and choking or gagging.
D. A breathing pattern that has 3 or more respiratory pauses longer than 3 seconds with less than 20 seconds of respiration between pauses.
E. A respiratory pause lasting more than 20 seconds. It may be associated with cyanosis, pallor, hypotonia, or bradycardia. A general term used to describe a condition in infants of any gestational age.

8. Causes of apnea may include:
   A. decreased oxygen delivery.
   B. cardiac arrhythmia.
   C. central nervous system disease.
   D. all of the above.

Questions 9 to 12: Match the types of apnea recordings in Column I with the selected indications in Column II. Use each answer ONCE.

Column I

9. Documented event monitoring
10. Pneumogram
11. Multichannel respiratory recording
12. Polysomnogram

Column II

A. To evaluate patient events or to verify the presence or absence of central apnea, bradycardia, or desaturation.
B. To monitor parameters of other multichannel recorders as well as EEG, EOG, and EMG.
C. To use airflow thermistry for the detection of central apnea, obstructive apnea, bradycardia, and oxygen desaturation.
D. To detect central apnea, obstructive apnea, bradycardia, and oxygen desaturation; to evaluate capnography, air flow or volume, and esophageal pH or pressure.

13. Among the following abnormal breathing patterns, _____ may be a normal event for some patients.
    A. periodic breathing
    B. central apnea
    C. obstructive apnea
    D. mixed apnea

14. The most common management techniques for infants with apnea include all of the following *except:*
    A. theophylline.
    B. albuterol.
    C. methylxanthine.
    D. caffeine.

15. Among the commonly used medications for the management of apnea, _____ should not be given at home because of its short half-life, need for frequent administration, and potential for toxicity.
    A. anticholinergic
    B. caffeine
    C. theophylline
    D. albuterol

Questions 16 to 19: Infant Jones is being sent home with an apnea monitor after staying in the neonatal intensive care unit (NICU) for over six weeks due to prematurity and occasional apneas.

16. You are assigned to assist in the discharge planning for infant Jones. You would ensure that at least one family member at home is able to do all of the following *except:*
    A. perform neonatal CPR.
    B. use the monitor properly to include the signals and alarms on the monitor.
    C. monitor and assess the infant when not at home and without the monitor.
    D. call 911 in case of monitor malfunction.

17. Prior to discharge, you are providing instructions to the family members on the use of an apnea monitor. You would include in your instructions that in the event that the alarms go off on an apnea monitor, the caretaker should first check the _____ and then the _____.
    A. monitor; infant
    B. type of alarm; infant
    C. infant; monitor
    D. infant; type of alarm

18. Regarding alarm episodes, you would instruct the family members that all of the following quick assessments should be done at home to evaluate the status of the infant *except:*
    A. development of hypotension.
    B. appearance of cyanosis.
    C. lack of chest movement.
    D. lack of air flow through the nose.

19. You would also instruct the family members that during a prolonged apnea episode, the caretaker should perform the following procedures in proper sequence (starting with the first step).
    I. Rubbing of back and tapping of sole of foot with loud vocal sounds
    II. Gentle stimulation
    III. CPR
    A. I, II, and III.
    B. I, III, and II
    C. II, I, and III
    D. II, III, and I

20. A family member asks you about the timing for discontinuation of the apnea monitor. You would tell him that the monitor could be discontinued when all of the following conditions are met *except:*
    A. a family member reports that the infant is breathing adequately.
    B. the infant is able to breathe adequately without respiratory stimulants.
    C. there are no significant clinical alarms for at least four weeks.
    D. normal values are documented from the monitor recorder.

CHAPTER 31 Medical Gases—Manufacture, Storage, and Delivery

1. Room air consists of about:
   A. 0.01% hydrogen.
   B. 0.03% carbon dioxide.
   C. 23% oxygen.
   D. 76% nitrogen.

2. The partial pressure of a gas is proportional to the:
   A. concentration of the gas in a mixture.
   B. barometric pressure.
   C. molecular weight of the gas.
   D. A and B only.

3. Given: F_IO_2 = 40%, P_B = 760 mm Hg. What is the partial pressure of oxygen in the inspired gas (P_IO_2) in a dry gas mixture?
   A. 19 mm Hg
   B. 30 mm Hg
   C. 190 mm Hg
   D. 304 mm Hg

4. The barometric pressure on Mount Elbert, CO, at 14,433 ft is 446 mm Hg. What is the F_IO_2 and partial pressure of oxygen in the inspired gas (P_IO_2) in a dry gas mixture?
   A. F_IO_2 = 10%; P_IO_2 = 9 mm Hg
   B. F_IO_2 = 15%; P_IO_2 = 32 mm Hg
   C. F_IO_2 = 21%; P_IO_2 = 94 mm Hg
   D. Insufficient information to calculate answer

5. Fractional distillation of liquefied air is the commercial process to produce:
   A. oxygen.
   B. nitrogen.
   C. carbon dioxide.
   D. compressed air.

6. Ms. Olson, a patient with COPD, is using oxygen at home via a concentrator. This machine produces oxygen using the process of:
   A. photosynthesis.
   B. molecular filtration.
   C. electrolysis of water.
   D. fractional distillation of air.

Questions 7 to 12: Match the gases in Column I with the most common clinical applications in Column II. Use each answer ONCE.

Column I

7. Oxygen (O_2)
8. Carbon dioxide (CO_2)
9. Helium (He)
10. Nitric oxide (NO)
11. Nitrous oxide (N_2O)
12. Nitrogen (N_2)

Column II

A. To treat persistent pulmonary hypertension of the newborn and other conditions characterized by hypoxemia and pulmonary hypertension
B. To power pneumatic instruments in the operating room
C. To use as an anesthetic
D. To calibrate capnographs, blood gas analyzers, and other laboratory equipment
E. To treat hypoxemia
F. To measure lung volumes; to mix with oxygen (helix therapy) for patients with airflow obstruction

13. _____ is the organization that provides safety standards governing cylinders, fittings, and connections.
   A. Compressed Gas Association (CGA)
   B. Department of Transportation (DOT)
   C. National Fire Protection Association (NFPA)
   D. International Standards Organization

14. The Department of Transportation (DOT) requires that gas cylinders be tested at regular intervals of every _____ years for steel cylinders and every _____ years for aluminum cylinders.
    A. 5; 10
    B. 10; 15
    C. 10; 5
    D. 15; 10

15. Hydrostatic testing is done by submerging the cylinder in water and pressurizing the cylinder to _____ greater than its normal filling pressure. The volume of expansion is measured by the amount of _____ displaced.
    A. two-thirds; air
    B. two-thirds; water
    C. three-fifths; air
    D. three-fifths; water

Questions 16 to 21: Match the type of gas in Column I with the respective U.S. color coding on cylinders in Column II. Use each answer ONCE.

Column I	Column II
16. Oxygen (O_2)	A. Brown
	B. Yellow
17. Carbon dioxide (CO_2)	C. Green
	D. Blue
18. Helium (He)	E. Gray
	F. Black
19. Nitrogen (N_2)	
20. Air	
21. Nitrous oxide (N_2O)	

22. Transfilling of a single small cylinder from a larger full cylinder is dangerous due to lack of a _____ to prevent rapid buildup of _____.
    A. flow limiter; heat
    B. flow limiter; pressure
    C. regulator; heat
    D. regulator; pressure

23. The indexed safety system for high-pressure cylinders size E and smaller is called:
    A. American Standard Safety System.
    B. Pin-Index Safety System.
    C. Diameter-Index Safety System.
    D. Compressed Gas Association System.

Questions 24 to 26. You are called to take part in a patient transport by helicopter. As you are checking the portable oxygen cylinders, you notice that one of the E-size cylinders reads 1000 psig.

24. With the information given above, how long would this cylinder with 1000 psig of compressed oxygen last if the required oxygen flow during the transport was 4 L/min?
    A. 25 min
    B. 40 min
    C. 70 min
    D. 250 min

25. With the information given above, would this cylinder contain enough oxygen for a one-way trip lasting 90 minutes?
    A. No at 4 L/min
    B. Yes at 4 L/min
    C. Yes at 5 L/min
    D. Not enough information to calculate answer

26. With the information given above, you would bring at least _____ cylinder(s) in the event that the patient had to return to the original destination (round-trip time = 3 hours).
    A. one
    B. two
    C. three
    D. four

27. How long would a full size K oxygen cylinder (2200 psig) last at a continuous flow rate of 5 L/min?
    A. 17 hours
    B. 19 hours
    C. 21 hours
    D. 23 hours

28. How long would a size K oxygen cylinder at 2200 psig last at a continuous flow rate of 5 L/min until the pressure drops to 500 psig?
    A. 17 hours, 47 min
    B. 19 hours, 22 min
    C. 21 hours, 35 min
    D. 23 hours, 11 min

29. Liquid oxygen is ideal for bulk storage because 1 L of liquid oxygen equals _____ L of gaseous oxygen.
    A. 8
    B. 86
    C. 861
    D. 8,610

30. Shut-off valves used in a gas piping system are designed for _____ reasons.
    A. business license
    B. insurance
    C. accreditation
    D. safety

31. At the patient's bedside, the working pressure for piped-in compressed air is _____, whereas the working pressure for a vacuum is _____.
    A. 10 to 20 psig; –10 to –40 mm Hg
    B. 10 to 20 psig; –20 to –200 mm Hg
    C. 50 to 55 psig; –10 to –40 mm Hg
    D. 50 to 55 psig; –20 to –200 mm Hg

CHAPTER 32 Oxygen Therapy: Administration and Management

1. Regulators are used to _____ the system gas pressure to a level suitable for the intended devices.
   A. increase
   B. reduce
   C. stop
   D. measure

2. Based on the AARC Clinical Practice Guideline, indications for oxygen therapy include all of the following *except*:
   A. hypoxemia.
   B. postanesthesia recovery.
   C. acute myocardial infarction.
   D. hypercapnia.

3. With downstream resistance or partial obstruction, the actual flow delivered by a Bourdon gauge is _____ the set flow rate as indicated on the gauge.
   A. higher than
   B. lower than
   C. same as
   D. unable to determine answer without an actual flow rate

4. With downstream resistance or partial obstruction, the actual flow delivered by a _____ Thorpe tube flowmeter is _____ the set flow rate as indicated on the flowmeter.
   A. pressure-compensated; the same as
   B. pressure-compensated; higher than
   C. nonpressure-compensated; the same as
   D. nonpressure-compensated; lower than

Questions 5 to 7: Match the types of common oxygen sources in Column I with the respective descriptions in Column II. Use each answer ONCE.

Column I	Column II
5. Oxygen concentrators	A. Gas pressure up to 2200 psig in common sizes of E and K
	B. Molecular absorption of nitrogen
6. Oxygen cylinders	C. Gas pressure of 22 psig in common capacities from 12 to 60 L
7. Liquid oxygen system	

8. In case of power failure, backup oxygen cylinders must be available if the patient is using a(n) _____ at home.
   A. size E oxygen cylinder
   B. oxygen concentrator
   C. liquid oxygen system
   D. all of the above

9. By definition, a high flow oxygen device is one that maintains a stable _____ and meets a patient's full inspiratory _____ requirement.
   A. flow; F_IO_2
   B. flow; tidal volume
   C. F_IO_2; flow
   D. F_IO_2; tidal volume

Questions 10 to 13: Match the oxygen adminis-
tering devices for adults in Column I with the
respective F$_I$O$_2$ range in Column II. Use each
answer ONCE.

Column I   Column II

10. Nasal cannula   A. 60% to 80% at flows of 10 to
                               15 L/min
11. Simple mask   B. 40% to 70% at flows of 8 to
                               15 L/min
12. Partial rebreathing   C. 24% to 40% at flows of 1 to
    mask   5 L/min
                            D. 30% to 60% at flows of 5 to
13. Non-rebreathing   10 L/min
    mask

14. When nasal oxygen cannula are used on infants, a flow
    of 0.25 L/min may produce an F$_I$O$_2$ of:
    A. 24%.
    B. 28%.
    C. 32%.
    D. 35%.

15. When a low flow oxygen device (e.g., nasal cannula) is
    used, the F$_I$O$_2$ depends on a user's:
    A. tidal volume.
    B. respiratory rate.
    C. dead space volume.
    D. all of the above.

16. When a low flow oxygen device is used, the F$_I$O$_2$ may
    be increased when the breathing pattern is:
    A. fast and shallow.
    B. fast and deep.
    C. slow and shallow.
    D. slow and deep.

17. The figure shown above represents a(n):
    A. simple oxygen face mask.
    B. partial-rebreathing mask.
    C. non-rebreathing mask.
    D. anesthesia mask.

18. You have just finished setting up a partial-rebreathing
    mask. How would you determine the initial oxygen
    flow?
    A. 10 L/min
    B. 15 L/min
    C. Sufficient to keep the bag partially inflated
       throughout inspiration
    D. Sufficient to keep the bag partially inflated
       throughout expiration

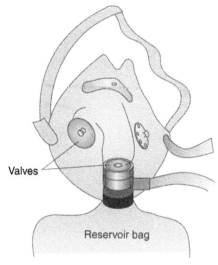

(Illustration modified from Scanlan CL, Wilkins RL, Stoller JK:
Egan's Fundamentals of respiratory care, ed 7, St. Louis, Mosby,
1999.)

19. Oxygen-conserving devices include all of the following
    except:
    A. reservoir cannula.
    B. demand-oxygen conserver.
    C. transtracheal catheter.
    D. Venturi mask.

20. Air-entrainment mask is a _____ oxygen device
    since it delivers a precise F$_I$O$_2$ and meets a user's
    _____ requirement.
    A. high-flow; inspiratory flow
    B. high-flow; tidal volume
    C. low-flow; inspiratory flow
    D. low-flow; tidal volume

Questions 21 to 24. Mr. Smith, one of your
patients in the surgical intensive care unit, is
using a 60% air-entrainment mask following
abdominal surgery.

21. As you are doing oxygen rounds, you notice that the
    air-entrainment port is unprotected by a shield and is
    covered by a blanket. This condition would:
    A. cause a higher F$_I$O$_2$.
    B. cause a lower F$_I$O$_2$.
    C. not affect the F$_I$O$_2$.
    D. cause the patient to hyperventilate.

22. What is the oxygen-to-air ratio for Mr. Smith's air-
    entrainment mask?
    A. 1:0.5
    B. 1:1
    C. 1:1.5
    D. 1:2

23. If the oxygen flow is set at 8 L/min for Mr. Smith's air-entrainment mask, what is the total flow?
    A. 10 L/min
    B. 12 L/min
    C. 14 L/min
    D. 16 L/min

24. If Mr. Smith has a peak inspiratory flow of 12 L/min during spontaneous breathing, would the air-entrainment mask setup meet his ventilatory needs? If not, what should be done?
    A. Yes
    B. No, the flow rate should be increased to 12 L/min
    C. No, the flow rate should be increased to 16 L/min
    D. Not enough information to determine answer

25. The oxygen device that covers a neonate's entire head is called a(n):
    A. tent.
    B. face mask.
    C. hood.
    D. incubator.

26. Polarographic and galvanic cell oxygen analyzers measure the _____ and they are calibrated using _____.
    A. F_IO_2; room air
    B. F_IO_2; room air or 100% oxygen
    C. pO_2; room air
    D. pO_2; room air or 100% oxygen

CHAPTER 33

Hyperbaric Oxygen

1. One atmospheric pressure equals:
   A. 50 pounds per square inch.
   B. 760 millimeters of mercury.
   C. 103 centimeters of water.
   D. 10 feet of water.

2. The atmospheric pressure for a diver who is 33 feet below the water surface is about:
   A. 760 mm Hg.
   B. 1000 mm Hg.
   C. 1520 mm Hg.
   D. 2280 mm Hg.

3. While breathing compressed air (21% oxygen), the P_IO_2 for a diver who is 33 feet below the water surface is about:
   A. 159 mm Hg.
   B. 210 mm Hg.
   C. 319 mm Hg.
   D. 693 mm Hg.

Questions 4 to 8: Match the "laws" in Column I with the respective descriptions in Column II. Use each answer ONCE.

Column I

4. Boyle's law

5. Charles' law

6. Gay-Lussac's law

7. Pascal's law

8. Henry's law

Column II

A. The pressure of a gas varies directly with the absolute temperature when the volume is kept constant.

B. The solubility of a gas in a liquid is directly proportional to the partial pressure of the gas over the liquid.

C. The pressure applied to an enclosed liquid is transmitted uniformly and undiminished to all parts of the liquid.

D. The volume of a gas varies directly with the absolute temperature when the pressure is kept constant.

E. The volume of a gas varies inversely with the pressure when the temperature is kept constant.

9. Barotrauma, inert gas narcosis, and oxygen toxicity are some problems that a person may encounter during gas _____ caused by _____ pressure.
   A. compression; increasing
   B. compression; decreasing
   C. decompression; increasing
   D. decompression; decreasing

10. Painful sensation in or around the joints is a sign of:
    A. type 1 compression sickness.
    B. type 1 decompression sickness.
    C. type 2 compression sickness.
    D. type 2 decompression sickness.

11. Arterial gas embolism is a problem encountered during _____ and the air may leak into the _____.
    A. compression; pleural space
    B. compression; pleural space, mediastinum, or brain
    C. decompression; pleural space
    D. decompression; pleural space, mediastinum, or brain

12. Ascending from a depth of 33 feet below the water surface, the diver must continually _____ because the lung volume is _____ during ascent.
    A. inhale and build up the lung volume; decreasing
    B. breathe normally; unchanged
    C. exhale and vent the extra gas volume; increasing
    D. hold his or her breath; unchanged

13. A diver is in the emergency room suffering from severe arterial gas embolism. To treat this condition, you would implement all of the following procedures *except:*
    A. chest tube.
    B. 50% oxygen.
    C. 50% nitrogen.
    D. compression to 6 atmospheric pressures.

14. Indications for hyperbaric oxygen therapy include all of the following *except:*
    A. carbon monoxide poisoning.
    B. emphysema with carbon dioxide retention.
    C. gas gangrene.
    D. air or gas embolism.

15. The absolute contraindication for hyperbaric oxygen therapy is:
    A. untreated pneumothorax.
    B. pregnancy.
    C. seizure disorder.
    D. air embolism.

16. Delivery of oxygen under pressure _____ the gas bubble size in the circulation and tissue, thus _____ circulation.
    A. increases; hindering
    B. increases; improving
    C. decreases; hindering
    D. decreases; improving

17. Delivery of oxygen under pressure inhibits growth of _____ and this technique is useful in many types of _____ care.
    A. anaerobes; respiratory
    B. anaerobes; wound
    C. aerobes; respiratory
    D. aerobes; wound

18. During hyperbaric oxygen therapy:
    A. cosmetics and jewelry should not be inside the chamber.
    B. oral and intravenous medications should not be administered.
    C. subcutaneous or intramuscular injections should not be given.
    D. antihypertensive drugs and neuromuscular relaxers should not be given.

19. The most common hyperbaric system is the class _____ chamber, which is for _____ occupancy.
    A. A; single
    B. A; multiple
    C. B; single
    D. B; multiple

20. During decompression, the temperature inside the chamber _____ in response to the physics of _____ law.
    A. increases; Boyle's
    B. increases; Charles'
    C. decreases; Dalton's
    D. decreases; Guy-Lussac's

21. _____ may be used during hyperbaric oxygen therapy.
    A. Microwave heated blanket
    B. Hand warmer
    C. Ventilator
    D. Sparking toys

22. Development of _____ during decompression in a single occupancy chamber is a serious problem because if decompression is allowed to continue, the problem will get worse.
    A. oxygen toxicity
    B. tension pneumothorax
    C. gas embolism
    D. decompression sickness

23. Since the volume varies with changing pressure, the cuff of an endotracheal tube should be _____ prior to hyperbaric oxygen therapy.
    A. filled with saline
    B. filled with 10 cc of extra air
    C. deflated
    D. inflated to minimal occlusion volume

24. The National Fire Protection Agency (NFPA) sets standards for all of the following *except:*
    A. oxygen delivery and control specifications inside hyperbaric chamber.
    B. ventilation controls for hyperbaric chamber.
    C. materials allowed within the hyperbaric chamber.
    D. purity of gas used in hyperbaric chamber.

CHAPTER 34

Humidity and Aerosol Therapy

1. Lack of adequate humidity in the inspired gas may lead to:
   A. increase of ciliary activity.
   B. decrease of mucus production.
   C. decrease of airway irritability.
   D. thickening of secretions.

2. The *isothermic saturation boundary* refers to the location in the airway or lung parenchyma that the humidity content reaches _____ mg/L at _____.
   A. 44; 25° C
   B. 44; 37° C
   C. 47; 25° C
   D. 47; 37° C

3. The isothermic saturation boundary may be compromised when the:
   A. environmental temperature or humidity drops.
   B. upper airway is bypassed by an artificial airway.
   C. spontaneous tidal volume is increased.
   D. all of the above.

4. The most effective method to improve the character and mobilization of thick secretions is _____ by _____.
   A. humidity therapy; humidifier
   B. bronchodilator therapy; small volume nebulizer
   C. chest physiotherapy; hand percussion
   D. systemic hydration; intravenous fluid

5. Cool humidity or aerosol is commonly used to treat upper airway inflammation (e.g., croup) because it promotes localized peripheral _____ and _____ swelling of the mucosa.
   A. vasodilation; increases
   B. vasodilation; reduces
   C. vasoconstriction; increases
   D. vasoconstriction; reduces

Questions 6 to 8: Match the devices for humidification in Column I with the respective descriptions in Column II. Use each answer ONCE.

Column I   Column II

6. Active humidifier   A. Adds water vapor or heat or both to the inspired gas
                          B. Produces aerosol or suspension of water particles in inspired gas
7. Passive humidifier   C. Uses exhaled moisture and heat to humidify inspired gas
8. Nebulizer

9. You are setting up a partial-rebreathing mask for a spontaneously breathing patient. The oxygen flow rate is at 8 L/min. You would use a:
   A. bubble humidifier.
   B. jet humidifier.
   C. heated bubble humidifier.
   D. passover humidifier.

10. A heated humidification system is intended for use in conjunction with a(n):
    A. nasal cannula.
    B. artificial airway.
    C. simple mask.
    D. non-rebreathing mask.

11. Water traps and heated wire circuits are used to minimize _____ in the tubing and contamination with _____.
    A. air flow resistance; bacteria
    B. air flow resistance; secretions
    C. condensation; bacteria
    D. condensation; secretions

Questions 12 to 14: Match the types of passive humidifiers in Column I with the construction material and percent efficiency in Column II. Use each answer ONCE.

Column I   Column II

12. Hygroscopic condenser humidifiers

13. Condenser humidifiers

14. Hydrophobic condenser humidifiers

A. Made with a water-repellent element with a large surface area and low thermal conductivity; 70% efficient

B. Made with metallic gauze, corrugated metal or parallel metal tubes that provide high thermal conductivity; 50% efficient

C. Made with materials that provide low thermal conductivity (e.g., paper, wool) impregnated with water-retaining chemical (e.g., calcium chloride or lithium chloride); 70% efficient

15. The efficiency of heat and moisture exchangers (HMEs) is reduced with:
    A. increasing tidal volume.
    B. increasing flow.
    C. increasing F_IO_2.
    D. all of the above.

16. In patients who are being mechanically ventilated, heat and moisture exchangers (HME) may increase the _____. This condition may be overcome by adding a low level of _____.
    A. compliance; pressure support
    B. compliance; positive end-expiratory pressure
    C. air flow resistance; pressure support
    D. air flow resistance; positive end-expiratory pressure

17. After assessing Mr. Varser, you are ready to start the in-line metered dose inhaler (MDI) therapy. Since he is using a heat and moisture exchanger (HME) while being mechanically ventilated, you would place the MDI attachment:
    A. on the expiratory limb of ventilator circuit.
    B. on the inspiratory limb of ventilator circuit.
    C. between the HME and the patient.
    D. between the HME and the ventilator circuit.

18. Mr. Hamlet, a patient who is being mechanically ventilated, has been producing copious amount of secretions. You would reevaluate whether the continuing use of _____ is appropriate for this patient.
    A. pressure support ventilation
    B. a heat and moisture exchanger
    C. an in-line suctioning device
    D. positive end-expiratory pressure

19. When a large-volume nebulizer (with air-entrainment capability) is used to deliver bland aerosol, the total flow is highest at this setting among which of the following?
    A. F_IO_2 = 24%, oxygen flow 4 L/min
    B. F_IO_2 = 30%, oxygen flow 8 L/min
    C. F_IO_2 = 40%, oxygen flow 10 L/min
    D. F_IO_2 = 60%, oxygen flow 15 L/min

Questions 20 to 24: Match the patient conditions in Column I with the appropriate humidification devices in Column II. Use each answer ONCE.

Column I   Column II

20. A patient who is being mechanically ventilated via an endotracheal tube

21. A patient using nasal cannula at 2 L/min oxygen

22. A patient who is breathing spontaneously via a fresh tracheal stoma and requires high humidity at 30% oxygen

23. A patient using a non-rebreathing mask at 15 L/min oxygen

A. No humidity is indicated.

B. Heated wick humidifier

C. Bubble humidifier

D. Large volume jet nebulizer with air-entrainment port

24. Deposition of aerosol particles in the lower respiratory tract is enhanced when the:
    A. tidal volume is low.
    B. aerosol droplets are in the 1 to 5 micron range.
    C. inspiratory flow is high.
    D. respiratory rate is high.

25. Waste of aerosol generated by the small-volume nebulizers may be minimized by using:
    A. reservoir tubing on the expiratory limb of nebulizer setup.
    B. a vented nebulizer system.
    C. a breath-actuated nebulizer.
    D. all of the above.

26. You have just received an order to start aerosol therapy with pentamidine. You would use a:
    A. large-volume nebulizer.
    B. small-volume nebulizer.
    C. nebulizer with one-way valves and expiratory filter.
    D. nebulizer with one-way valves and inspiratory filter.

27. Aerosol delivery is most efficient when the therapy is administered to a(n):
    A. crying child.
    B. adult using an aerosol mask.
    C. adult breathing through the mouth.
    D. infant via blow-by technique.

28. During shift report, you are informed that a child in the pediatric unit is using a small particle aerosol generator (SPAG). You would reason that the child was receiving:
    A. pentamidine.
    B. ribavirin.
    C. continuous albuterol.
    D. acetylcysteine.

29. Mr. Farland, a 30-year-old patient in the emergency department, has an admitting diagnosis of acute exacerbation of asthma. The attending physician asks you to evaluate the patient and start bronchodilator therapy. You would use:
    A. 1 mg of albuterol via small-volume nebulizer.
    B. 10 mg of albuterol via small-volume nebulizer.
    C. continuous albuterol aerosol therapy 1 mg/hour.
    D. continuous albuterol aerosol therapy 10 mg/hour.

30. Overhydration and bronchospasm are two potential complications of:
    A. pressurized metered dose inhaler.
    B. heated bubble humidifier.
    C. ultrasonic nebulizer.
    D. small-volume aerosol therapy.

31. The most important aspect of using pressurized metered dose inhalers (pMDI) is:
    A. proper technique.
    B. storage temperature of inhaler.
    C. expiration date of inhaler.
    D. compliance with the frequency of use.

32. In regard to pressurized metered dose inhalers (pMDI), all of the following statements are correct *except:*
    A. pMDI can be repeated immediately after the first actuation.
    B. new pMDI should be actuated several times before first use.
    C. pMDI should be stored with the cap on.
    D. number of doses remaining should be recorded consistently.

33. A valved holding chamber is an accessory device that helps to _____ while using pMDI.
    A. reduce the need for hand-breath coordination
    B. reduce the size of aerosol particles
    C. increase deposition of some medications
    D. increase oropharyngeal deposition of drug

34. Dr. Holland asks you to instruct her patient on the use of dry powder inhaler (DPI). You would emphasize to the patient:
    A. that DPI must be used with a spacer.
    B. that DPI is dependent on inspiratory flow.
    C. to inhale as slowly as possible.
    D. to exhale back into the DPI device.

35. Rotahaler, Diskhaler, Diskus, and Turbuhaler are devices that deliver _____ medication.
    A. diuretic
    B. cardiac
    C. dry powder
    D. intravenous

36. The techniques used to deliver aerosolized bronchodilators during mechanical ventilation include all of the following *except:*
    A. nebulizer should be at least 30 cm from the patient Y-piece.
    B. nebulizer should be cleaned with sterile water, rinsed, and air dried after use.
    C. tidal volume should be 500 mL or higher for adults.
    D. pressure support should be set at 30 cm H_2O.

37. You are getting ready to administer pressurized metered dose inhaler (pMDI) to a patient who is being mechanically ventilated. You would follow all of the following techniques *except:*
    A. place the heat and moisture exchanger (HME) between the pMDI and patient Y-piece.
    B. minimize the inspiratory air flow during administration of pMDI.
    C. actuate the pMDI at the onset of mechanical breath.
    D. shake the pMDI canister vigorously prior to use.

CHAPTER 35

Secretion Clearance Techniques

1. In the ciliated epithelium of the airway, the gel layer has the ability to trap and hold:
   A. dust.
   B. pollens.
   C. microorganisms.
   D. all of the above.

2. The most essential factor in producing an effective cough is:
   A. high inspiratory flow.
   B. high expiratory flow.
   C. slow respiratory rate.
   D. fast respiratory rate.

3. In patients with COPD, coughs are not effective due to all of the following factors *except:*
   A. early airway closure on exhalation.
   B. reduced expiratory flow.
   C. large tidal volume.
   D. poor respiratory muscles and mechanics.

4. A patient asks you about the rationale of performing postural drainage. You would explain to him that it facilitates removal of secretions by the action of:
   A. gravity.
   B. vibration.
   C. dissociation.
   D. ionization.

5. The most effective method in loosening the dried secretions is to provide humidity via:
   A. aerosol therapy.
   B. humidity therapy.
   C. systemic hydration.
   D. hypertonic saline administration.

6. When *hypertonic* saline solution is administered via a nebulizer to the mucosa of airway, it causes movement of water from:
   A. secretion to airway.
   B. airway to secretion.
   C. airway to interstitial space.
   D. interstitial space to airway.

7. Acetylcysteine:
   A. is the generic name for Proventil.
   B. has a pleasant smell and taste.
   C. is used as a bronchodilator.
   D. is a mucolytic agent.

8. Which of the following statements is true in regard to aspiration (suctioning) of secretions by vacuum?
   A. Preoxygenation reduces sputum production.
   B. Prolonged suction may lead to hyperventilation.
   C. Suctioning may be done for up to 45 seconds.
   D. Routine saline administration should not be done.

9. Indications for nasotracheal suctioning include all of the following *except:*
   A. pneumonia.
   B. poor cough efforts.
   C. inability to clear secretions.
   D. audible evidence of secretions in large airways.

10. Contraindications for nasotracheal suctioning include all of the following *except:*
    A. occluded nasal passages.
    B. nasal bleeding.
    C. epiglottitis.
    D. bradycardia.

11. Indications for postural drainage are mainly limited to patients who produce more than _____ mL of secretions per day and have difficulty clearing the secretions.
    A. 5
    B. 10
    C. 30
    D. 300

12. "Shaking loose" the pulmonary secretions is the purpose of:
    A. postural drainage.
    B. percussion.
    C. huff coughing.
    D. manually assisted coughing.

13. Contraindications for postural drainage and percussion include all of the following conditions *except:*
    A. intracranial pressure greater than 5 mm Hg.
    B. pulmonary tuberculosis.
    C. osteoporosis and osteomyelitis of the ribs.
    D. risk for aspiration.

14. Postural drainage and percussion may be administered with extreme caution to patients with all of the following conditions *except:*
    A. pulmonary hemorrhage.
    B. COPD.
    C. hypoxemia.
    D. hypotension.

15. You are teaching secretion clearance techniques to a patient who has poor coughing efforts. In your coughing instruction, you would outline the proper sequence of an effective cough as follows:
    I. Hold breath by closing glottis.
    II. Take in deep breath.
    III. Release breath forcefully.
    IV. Build up pressure in lungs.
    A. I, II, IV, III
    B. I, IV, III, II
    C. II, I, IV, III
    D. II, IV, III, I

16. _____ is done by providing thrusts with hands and arms positioned on the patient's abdomen during exhalation.
    A. Huff coughing
    B. Manually assisted coughing
    C. Autogenic drainage
    D. Active cycle of breathing

17. Incentive spirometry:
    A. relies on a patient's effort to obtain maximum lung expansion.
    B. is the only therapy to treat atelectasis.
    C. should not be used as prophylactic therapy for postoperative atelectasis.
    D. should be used in patients with vital capacities less than 5 mL/Kg.

18. You are administering an IPPB therapy to Mr. Jones, a patient with severe atelectasis who has not had an IPPB therapy before. Following instructions Mr. Jones, you would adjust and fine-tune the _____ control on the IPPB machine until the expired volume is at least _____% larger than the patient's tidal volume.
    A. volume; 15
    B. volume; 25
    C. pressure; 15
    D. pressure; 25

19. The effectiveness of an IPPB therapy may be assessed by all of the following techniques *except:*
    A. improved secretion clearance.
    B. breath sounds.
    C. blood gases.
    D. chest radiography.

Questions 20 to 22: Match the types of positive airway pressure techniques in Column I with the respective characteristics in Column II. Use each answer ONCE.

Column I	Column II
20. Continuous positive airway pressure (CPAP)	A. Positive pressure (10 to 20 cm H$_2$O) in the airway during expiratory phase, generated as a patient exhales through a *fixed orifice* resistor
21. Positive expiratory pressure (PEP)	B. Positive pressure in the air way during expiratory phase, generated by a *threshold* resistor
22. Expiratory positive airway pressure (EPAP)	C. Application of positive pressure (5 to 20 cm H$_2$O) in the airway throughout a spontaneous breathing cycle

23. You are asked to provide instruction to Ms. Holland, a COPD patient who is using positive expiratory pressure (PEP) therapy for the first time. In your instruction, you would include all of the following key points *except:*
    A. choose and use a PEP resistor that can provide between 10 to 20 cm H_2O of pressure.
    B. breathe in through a one-way valve to a level larger than tidal volume but not to total lung capacity (TLC) level.
    C. actively exhale to functional residual capacity (FRC) level.
    D. use an I:E ratio of 1:1 to 1:2.

24. _____ is a pipe-shaped device that has a steel ball in the bowl which provides about 10 cm H_2O of pressure during exhalation.
    A. Flutter valve
    B. Percussionaire
    C. Hayek oscillator
    D. ThAIRapy Vest

CHAPTER 36

Airway Management

1. An oropharyngeal airway may be used to maintain a patent airway during _____ ventilation.
   A. spontaneous
   B. manual bag-mask
   C. mouth to tube
   D. all of the above

2. An oropharyngeal airway should not be used in a _____ patient because of the risk of _____.
   A. semi-comatose or an alert; aspiration
   B. comatose; hypoventilation
   C. comatose; aspiration
   D. semi-comatose or an alert; hypoventilation

3. An oropharyngeal airway may be inserted using a _____-degree approach and then rotating until reaching a resting position that provides unobstructed breathing.
   A. 90
   B. 90 or 180
   C. 180
   D. 180 or 270

4. Complications of oropharyngeal airways include all of the following *except:*
   A. hyperventilation.
   B. dental damage.
   C. airway obstruction.
   D. vomiting and aspiration.

Questions 5 to 8. You are called to the emergency department to insert an airway. The patient is alert and spontaneously breathing following a motorcycle accident. There are apparent external injuries to the face and mouth. The emergency department physician, Dr. Brumback, does not want to maneuver the mouth until facial radiography can be made.

5. Dr. Brumback asks you to insert a temporary airway until further evaluation can be made. You would use a(n):
   A. nasopharyngeal airway.
   B. oropharyngeal airway.
   C. endotracheal tube.
   D. laryngeal mask airway.

6. In order to select an airway that is appropriate for the patient, you would measure the distance from the patient's _____ to the meatus (opening) of the _____.
   A. nose; eye
   B. nose; ear
   C. chin; eye
   D. chin; ear

7. Prior to inserting this airway, you would lubricate it with:
   A. normal saline.
   B. lidocaine cream.
   C. water-soluble gel.
   D. sterile water.

8. After inserting the airway, you would inform Dr. Brumback and the emergency department staff that this airway may also be used to provide an access for:
   A. a suction catheter.
   B. a bronchoscope.
   C. oxygen therapy.
   D. all of the above.

9. Which of the following is not an indication for endotracheal intubation?
   A. Mask CPAP
   B. Prevention of aspiration
   C. Removal of secretions
   D. Mechanical ventilation

10. During your intubation rotation in the operating room, the anesthesiologist tells you that the patient is a class IV case based on visualization of airway structure during direct laryngoscopy. You would know that this is a(n) _____ intubation.
    A. very difficult
    B. moderately difficult
    C. easy
    D. very easy

Questions 11 to 14: Match the complicating factors for intubation in Column I with the examples in Column II. Use each answer ONCE.

Column I

Column II

11. Distorted anatomy

12. Inadequate neck mobility

13. Inadequate jaw mobility

14. Disproportionate soft tissues

A. Degenerative cervical arthritis
B. Temporomandibular joint (TMJ) dysfunction
C. Oversized tongue
D. Deviated larynx or trachea

15. The space between the vocal cords is called the _____ and it is the narrowest point of the upper airway in _____.
    A. tracheal ring; adults
    B. tracheal ring; children
    C. glottis; adults
    D. glottis; children

16. The _____ of an endotracheal tube allows visualization of the tube on radiographies.
    A. Murphy eye
    B. radiopaque line
    C. cuff
    D. pilot balloon

Questions 17 to 23. You are paged to the medical intensive care unit to perform an elective intubation on Mr. Dawson, a patient with COPD and pneumonia. He is breathing spontaneously and is developing respiratory muscle fatigue. The physician wants to rest him on mechanical ventilation.

17. Mr. Dawson is 45 years old, 5'3", and 80 Kg. You would select and use a size _____ endotracheal tube.
    A. 6
    B. 7
    C. 8
    D. 9

18. Besides the endotracheal tube, which of the following supplies is optional and not required to complete the intubation procedure successfully?
    A. 10-cc syringe
    B. Stylet
    C. Laryngoscope handle
    D. Laryngoscope blade

19. After attaching the MacIntosh blade to the handle, the proper technique is to place the tip of the blade:
    A. at the base of the tongue.
    B. in the esophagus.
    C. in the vallecula.
    D. all of the above.

20. Since Mr. Dawson has a rather short neck, you decide to use a Miller blade instead. For this setup, the proper technique is to the tip of the blade until it is:
    A. able to lift the tip of epiglottis.
    B. in the vallecula.
    C. at the base of the tongue.
    D. in the esophagus.

View of the glottis with the laryngoscope in the vallecula.

21. Referring to the figure shown above, _____ represents the vocal cords—an important landmark for endotracheal intubation.
    A. A
    B. B
    C. C
    D. D

22. To ensure successful intubation, you would pass the endotracheal tube through the _____ under direct vision.
    A. epiglottis
    B. larynx
    C. vocal cords
    D. base of the tongue

23. To ensure proper placement of the endotracheal tube, you would pass the tube _____ below the level of vocal cords and then confirm its placement by

    _____.
    A. 2 to 4 cm; auscultation
    B. 2 to 4 cm; auscultation and chest radiography
    C. 2 to in; auscultation
    D. 2 to in; auscultation and chest radiography

24. Before the chest radiography is ready for final determination of tube position, the endotracheal tube may be secured near the _____ cm mark at Mr. Dawson's

    _____.
    A. 18 to 20; lips
    B. 18 to 20; teeth
    C. 21 to 23; lips
    D. 21 to 23; teeth

25. Laryngeal mask airway consists of a large-bore tube with a small, _____ mask at its distal end that forms a seal around the _____ opening.
    A. noninflatable; glottic
    B. noninflatable; esophageal
    C. inflatable; glottic
    D. inflatable; esophageal

26. Stridor is a complication of intubation that occurs:
    A. during the intubation procedure.
    B. while the endotracheal tube is in place.
    C. immediately following extubation.
    D. a long time after extubation.

27. Ideally, the distal end of an endotracheal tube should be _____ above the carina.
    A. 1 to 4 cm
    B. 3 to 7 cm
    C. 7 to 10 cm
    D. at least 10 cm

28. Comparing an endotracheal tube and a tracheostomy tube, the
    A. endotracheal tube allows a patient to swallow.
    B. endotracheal tube has a higher risk of infection.
    C. tracheostomy tube is better tolerated by the patient.
    D. tracheostomy tube carries lower surgical risks.

29. An uncuffed tracheostomy tube or uncuffed endotracheal tube is used in _____ patients because the _____ serves as an anatomic seal.
    A. pediatric; cricoid ring
    B. pediatric; glottis
    C. adult; cricoid ring
    D. adult; glottis

30. While using a fenestrated tracheostomy tube, a patient may talk and breathe spontaneously with the:
    I. proximal end of tube occluded.
    II. cuff deflated.
    III. cuff inflated.
    IV. inner cannula of tube removed.
    A. I and II
    B. I, II, and IV
    C. I, III, and IV
    D. III and IV

31. Dr. Goodnow asks you to instruct a patient on the use of the Passy-Muir tracheostomy speaking valve. You would include which of the following in your instruction?
    I. The valve works only during mechanical ventilation.
    II. The cuff must be inflated during use.
    III. The cuff must be deflated during use.
    IV. The valve eliminates the need for finger occlusion to speak.
    A. I and II
    B. I, II, and IV
    C. I, III, and IV
    D. III and IV

Questions 32 to 33: During ICU rounds, you notice that the patient is making vocal sounds while receiving mechanical ventilation. After assessing the patient-ventilator system, you conclude that the cuff needs to be inflated.

32. Since you cannot find the cuff pressure manometer immediately, you would manage the cuff by using the _____ technique and then go look for a cuff manometer.
    A. sniff position
    B. maximal inflation volume
    C. minimum occlusion pressure
    D. 10-cc syringe

33. After finding a cuff manometer, you would inflate the cuff between _____ mm Hg and reassess the patient.
    A. 10 to 15 mm Hg
    B. 20 to 25 mm Hg
    C. 30 to 35 mm Hg
    D. 40 to 45 mm Hg

34. Endotracheal suctioning should be done:
    A. at least once per shift.
    B. q 4 hours.
    C. QID.
    D. as needed.

35. Endotracheal suctioning should not be done at a regular interval because excessive suctioning may cause:
    A. bronchospasm.
    B. transient hypoxemia.
    C. suction-related atelectasis.
    D. all of the above.

36. Mr. Jones, a 60-year-old patient, has been producing a copious amount of secretions in the endotracheal tube. After assessing the patient, you determine that suctioning is indicated. You would use a size _____ suction catheter and adjust the suction pressure at _____ mm Hg.
    A. 14; 100
    B. 14; 150
    C. 18; 100
    D. 18; 150

37. During prolonged endotracheal suctioning, suction-related hypoxemia may lead to _____, whereas vagal stimulation may cause _____.
    A. arrhythmias; bradycardia
    B. arrhythmias; tachycardia
    C. bradycardia; arrhythmias
    D. tachycardia; arrhythmias

38. Your department has just started using the closed suction catheters and the department head asks you to establish the change-out frequency. Based on available literature and clinical evidence, you would suggest changing these catheters:
    A. twice per day.
    B. once per day.
    C. once every three days.
    D. once per week.

39. Before extubation, the patient must meet all of the following conditions *except*:
    A. ventilate without mechanical ventilation.
    B. ventilate without supplemental oxygen.
    C. keep a patent airway.
    D. clear secretions.

40. All of the following devices may be used to assess a patient's ability to use the upper airway and breathe without a tracheostomy tube *except*:
    A. smaller tracheostomy tube.
    B. cuffless endotracheal tube.
    C. Passy-Muir valve.
    D. cuffed endotracheal tube.

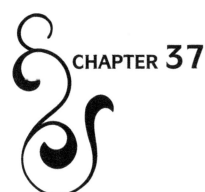

CHAPTER 37

Cardiopulmonary Resuscitation

1. Cardiopulmonary resuscitation is performed when the patient goes into:
   A. cardiac arrest.
   B. respiratory arrest.
   C. drug overdose.
   D. A or B.

2. During cardiopulmonary resuscitation, you are asked to perform defibrillation. You would evaluate the cardiac monitor and defibrillate for all of the following conditions *except:*
   A. cardiac arrest.
   B. ventricular fibrillation.
   C. premature ventricular contractions.
   D. pulseless ventricular tachycardia.

3. The first action in basic or advanced life support is to establish or initiate:
   A. an airway.
   B. breathing.
   C. circulation.
   D. defibrillation.

4. Dr. Samford asks you to establish an airway for a patient who has been brought to the emergency department following a motor vehicle accident. The patient has a cervical collar with possible cervical spine injury. You would manage the patient using the:
   A. jaw-thrust maneuver.
   B. head-tilt technique.
   C. chin-lift technique.
   D. Sellick maneuver.

5. Establishment of an airway with an endotracheal tube offers all of the following advantages for resuscitation *except:*
   A. provide ventilation and oxygenation.
   B. prevent gastric insufflation.
   C. obtain sputum samples.
   D. administer cardiac drugs in lack of intravenous access.

6. Following intubating a patient in the emergency department, you may verify the proper placement of the endotracheal tube by auscultation and:
   A. presence of CO_2 in expired gas.
   B. rising SPO_2 reading.
   C. inflation of the bulb attached to the endotracheal tube.
   D. any of the above.

7. A pharyngotracheal lumen (PTL) airway has _____ lumen(s) and it is placed in the patient's _____.
   A. one; esophagus
   B. one; esophagus or trachea
   C. two; trachea
   D. two; trachea or esophagus

8. An Esophageal-Tracheal Combitube (ETC) airway has _____ tube(s) and it is placed in the patient's _____.
   A. one; esophagus
   B. one; esophagus or trachea
   C. two; trachea
   D. two; trachea or esophagus

9. The _____ has a small mask on the distal end of the tube and it is inflated to provide a seal around the base of the tongue and the glottis.
   A. Esophageal-Tracheal Combitube
   B. laryngeal mask airway
   C. esophageal obturator airway
   D. pharyngotracheal lumen airway

10. During adult cardiopulmonary resuscitation, ventilation should be provided at a rate of _____ per minute and a volume from _____ with supplemental oxygen.
    A. 10 to 12; 400 to 600 mL
    B. 10 to 12; 700 to 1000 mL
    C. 14 to 16; 400 to 600 mL
    D. 14 to 16; 700 to 1000 mL

11. During adult cardiopulmonary resuscitation, cardiac compression should be provided at a depth of _____ inches and a rate of _____ per minute.
    A. 1.5 to 2; 60
    B. 1.5 to 2; 100
    C. 2 to 2.5; 100
    D. 2 to 2.5; 120

12. During adult cardiopulmonary resuscitation, the recommended cardiac compression-to-ventilation ratio is _____ before intubation and _____ after intubation.
    A. 5:1; 10:2
    B. 5:1; 15:2
    C. 10:2; 5:1
    D. 15:2; 5:1

13. The automatic external defibrillator (AED):
    A. does not offer analysis of cardiac rhythm.
    B. is attached to the patient via one adhesive pad via connecting cable.
    C. is used in cardiac arrest situations.
    D. is available for use in the hospital only.

14. The Heimlich maneuver is used to:
    A. facilitate endotracheal intubation.
    B. relieve upper airway obstruction.
    C. assist cardiopulmonary resuscitation.
    D. prevent aspiration.

15. During cardiopulmonary resuscitation of a child, cardiac compression should be provided at a depth of _____ inches and a rate of _____ per minute.
    A. 1 to 1.5; 60
    B. 1 to 1.5; 100
    C. 1.5 to 2; 60
    D. 1.5 to 2; 100

16. During cardiopulmonary resuscitation of an infant, cardiac compression should be provided at a depth of _____ inches and a rate of _____ per minute.
    A. 0.5 to 1; at least 100
    B. 0.5 to 1; no more than 100
    C. 1 to 1.5; at least 100
    D. 1 to 1.5; no more than 100

17. When drugs are administered via the endotracheal tube, the dosage used should be _____ times the intravenous dose diluted in _____ mL of normal saline.
    A. 2; 10
    B. 2; 20
    C. 5; 10
    D. 5; 20

Questions 18 to 20. You are called to the emergency department for an incoming cardiac arrest victim. The 40-year-old patient, Mr. Smith, is orally intubated. Cardiopulmonary resuscitation has been ongoing for 15 minutes in the ambulance.

18. During CPR in the emergency department, the cardiac rhythm shows asystole. Dr. Fellows asks you to defibrillate Mr. Smith. You would deliver the initial shock with _____ joules.
    A. 100
    B. 150
    C. 200
    D. 300

19. After the initial shock, the cardiac rhythm is changed to ventricular fibrillation. Dr. Fellows asks you to defibrillate again. You would deliver the second shock with _____ joules.
    A. 200
    B. 300
    C. 360
    D. 400

20. After the second defibrillation attempt, ventricular fibrillation persists. You would deliver the third shock with _____ joules.
    A. 200
    B. 300
    C. 360
    D. 400

Questions 21 to 25: Match the ACLS drugs in Column I with the respective indications in Column II. Review all options before answering these questions as indications may overlap. Use each answer ONCE.

Column I	Column II
21. Epinephrine	A. Ischemic chest pain, CHF
	B. Acute pulmonary edema, fluid overload
22. Dopamine	C. First drug in cardiac arrest
	D. Hypotension, cardiogenic shock
23. Atropine	E. Bradycardia
24. Furosemide	
25. Morphine sulfate	

CHAPTER 38

Pulmonary Rehabilitation

1. For patients with COPD, exercise training in a pulmonary rehabilitation program is effective to:
   I. increase the exercise capacity.
   II. improve the psychologic state.
   III. improve the pulmonary function.
   A. I and II.
   B. I and III.
   C. II and III.
   D. I, II, and III.

2. In addition to damage to lung tissue and airways, chronic lung disease can cause an increase in:
   A. pulmonary reserve.
   B. pulmonary vascular resistance.
   C. exercise tolerance.
   D. psychological well-being.

3. Mr. King, a patient in the pulmonary rehabilitation program, has a history of exertional dyspnea. This means that he is feeling short of breath:
   A. at rest.
   B. at bedtime.
   C. while performing physical work.
   D. around the clock.

4. Exercise training, education, medication optimization, bronchial hygiene, and psychosocial support are components of a(n) _____ rehabilitation program.
   A. intensive pulmonary
   B. maintenance pulmonary
   C. intensive cardiac
   D. maintenance cardiac

5. Supervised home program, exercise conditioning, and support group are vital components of a(n) _____ rehabilitation program.
   A. intensive pulmonary
   B. maintenance pulmonary
   C. intensive cardiac
   D. maintenance cardiac

6. Pulmonary rehabilitation program may be suitable for an individual:
   A. with stable chronic respiratory disease.
   B. who experiences exertional dyspnea.
   C. who is symptomatic.
   D. all of the above.

7. A multidisciplinary pulmonary rehabilitation program may be suitable for patients with any of the following conditions *except:*
   A. restrictive lung disease.
   B. congestive heart failure.
   C. transplantation.
   D. lung reduction surgery.

8. Hypercapnic COPD patients should be _____ a pulmonary rehabilitation program because they tend to tolerate exercise _____.
   A. included in; well with appropriate medications
   B. included in; well
   C. excluded from; poorly regardless of medications used
   D. excluded from; poorly

9. Exercise assessment is done prior to enrolling a patient into a rehabilitation program because it helps to:
   A. establish the initial exercise loads for patients.
   B. define program expectations for patients.
   C. focus specific therapies to be performed by patients.
   D. all of the above.

10. Five minutes into exercise assessment, the patient's SpO_2 level drops below 85%. However, there are no signs of bronchospasm. From these findings, you would include _____ as part of the patient's rehabilitation program.
    A. treadmill
    B. oxygen therapy
    C. bronchodilator therapy
    D. stationary bicycle

11. During patient assessment and visit with family members, you find that a patient has been rather inactive and isolated from social and family events. From these findings, you would recommend _____ in order to evaluate the patient's needs in a rehabilitation program.
    A. psychosocial assessment
    B. complete laboratory testing
    C. family counseling sessions
    D. support group sessions

12. Depending on a patient's specific needs, all of the following should be considered as part of patient assessment *except:*
    A. physical and occupational therapy evaluations.
    B. assessment of the patient's financial and insurance coverage.
    C. activities of daily living (ADL) evaluations.
    D. assessment of the patient's knowledge of the disease process.

13. In order to document the patient's competency on the use of metered-dose inhalers, _____ should be used as part of the educational process.
    A. written tests
    B. lecture
    C. demonstration and return demonstration
    D. discussion

14. _____ are most suitable for educating a patient about the disease process.
    A. Lecture and discussion
    B. Demonstration and return demonstration
    C. Written tests
    D. Practice sessions

Questions 15 to 17: Match the types of exercise in Column I with the purpose or training strategy in Column II. Use each answer ONCE.

Column I	Column II
15. Stretching and flexibility exercises	A. Uses a high-intensity and low-frequency strategy
16. Endurance exercises	B. Improves range of motion, provides general warm-up
17. Strengthening exercises	C. Uses a low-intensity and high-frequency strategy

18. Significant improvement in exercise performance and state of well-being may be found when _____ is part of the comprehensive exercise program for patients with COPD.
    A. arm exercise
    B. leg exercise
    C. arm and leg exercise
    D. breathing exercise

19. Dr. Johns has ordered strength training for a patient's upper extremities. You would select from all of the following devices *except:*
    A. treadmill.
    B. cross-country ski machine.
    C. free weights.
    D. rowing machine.

20. During each exercise session, the:
    A. patient should not use supplemental oxygen.
    B. patient should not take rest periods.
    C. workloads must be higher than the previous session.
    D. workloads should be reassessed and adjusted accordingly.

21. In endurance training, the patient should exercise _____ times per week and at least _____ minutes per exercise session.
    A. 3; 20
    B. 3; 30
    C. 5; 10
    D. 5; 20

22. During exercise, the patient's SpO_2 drops to 84%. You would:
    A. terminate the exercise program for the day.
    B. let the patient rest and resume exercise after 10 minutes.
    C. provide supplemental oxygen until SpO_2 during exercise is >88%.
    D. administer bronchodilator therapy as soon as possible.

23. Supplemental oxygen during exercise helps a patient to perform the exercise routines at a _____ duration and _____ intensity.
    A. longer; higher
    B. longer; lower
    C. shorter; higher
    D. shorter; lower

24. Pulmonary rehabilitation has been proven effective in *reducing* a patient's:
    A. sensation of shortness of breath.
    B. oxygen saturation.
    C. exercise tolerance.
    D. quality of life.

25. Pulmonary rehabilitation has been proven effective in *increasing* a patient's:
    A. sensation of shortness of breath.
    B. medical costs.
    C. exercise tolerance.
    D. health care use.

CHAPTER 39 Mechanical Ventilators: Classification and Principles of Operation

1. The most common input power sources for mechanical ventilators in the United States include all of the following *except:*
   A. 110 to 115 volts alternate current.
   B. rechargeable batteries.
   C. generators.
   D. compressed oxygen.

Questions 2 to 6

Resistance = Change in transairway pressure/change in flow

2. Based on the equation, all of the following statements are correct *except:*
   A. resistance is directly related to transairway pressure.
   B. resistance is inversely related to flow.
   C. flow is directly related to transairway pressure.
   D. flow is inversely related to transairway pressure.

3. At a constant transairway pressure, an increase in resistance would:
   A. have no effect on flow.
   B. increase the flow.
   C. decrease the flow.
   D. Insufficient information to determine answer

4. If a patient maintains the same level of work of breathing (constant transairway pressure), a condition such as asthma (increase in resistance) would:
   A. have no effect on flow.
   B. increase the flow.
   C. decrease the flow.
   D. Insufficient information to determine answer

5. At a constant resistance, an increase in transairway pressure would:
   A. have no effect on flow.
   B. increase the flow.
   C. decrease the flow.
   D. Insufficient information to determine answer

6. If the condition of a patient's airway remains unchanged (constant resistance), an increase in the work of breathing (increase in transairway pressure) would:
   A. have no effect on flow.
   B. increase the flow.
   C. decrease the flow.
   D. Insufficient information to determine answer

Questions 7 to 11. See Figure 39-1 in textbook and refer to this equation: Elastance = Change in transthoracic pressure/change in volume

7. Based on the above equation, all of the following statements are correct *except:*
   A. elastance is directly related to transthoracic pressure.
   B. elastance is inversely related to volume.
   C. volume is directly related to transthoracic pressure.
   D. volume is inversely related to transthoracic pressure.

8. At a constant transthoracic pressure, an increase in elastance (decrease in compliance) would:
   A. have no effect on volume.
   B. increase the volume.
   C. decrease the volume.
   D. Insufficient information to determine answer

9. If the patient or ventilator maintains the same level of work of breathing (constant transthoracic pressure), a condition such as atelectasis (increase in elastance or decrease in compliance) would:
   A. have no effect on volume.
   B. increase the volume.
   C. decrease the volume.
   D. Insufficient information to determine answer

10. At a constant elastance, an increase in transthoracic pressure would:
    A. have no effect on volume.
    B. increase the volume.
    C. decrease the volume.
    D. Insufficient information to determine answer

11. If the condition of a patient's lung and thorax remains unchanged (constant elastance), an increase in the work of breathing (increase in transthoracic pressure) would:
    A. have no effect on volume.
    B. increase the volume.
    C. decrease the volume.
    D. Insufficient information to determine answer

Questions 12 to 13. Refer to the equation of motion:
Ventilator pressure = (elastance x volume) + (resistance x flow)

12. The ventilator pressure is:
    A. directly related to elastance.
    B. directly related to resistance.
    C. directly related to compliance.
    D. A and B.

13. In order to provide a constant volume or flow, the ventilator pressure must be increased in conditions of:
    A. increasing elastance.
    B. increasing resistance.
    C. increasing compliance.
    D. A or B.

14. During a ventilator-assisted breath, you notice that the pressure waveform remains constant as the patient's compliance and resistance change. This variable makes the ventilator a:
    A. pressure-limited ventilator.
    B. pressure controller.
    C. pressure-cycled ventilator.
    D. volume controller.

15. Since the unit for elastance is _____ and the unit for volume is L, the product of elastance and volume is _____.
    A. cm H_2O/L; cm H_2O
    B. cm H_2O/L; L
    C. cm H_2O; cm H_2O/L
    D. L; cm H_2O/L

16. Since the unit for resistance is _____ and the unit for flow is L/sec, the product of resistance and flow is _____.
    A. cm H_2O/L/sec; cm H_2O
    B. cm H_2O/L/sec; L
    C. cm H_2O; cm H_2O/L/sec
    D. L; cm H_2O/L/sec

17. The product of elastance and volume is _____ and the product of resistance and flow is _____.
    A. pressure; flow
    B. pressure; pressure
    C. volume; flow
    D. volume; pressure

18. When a ventilator uses two controllers (e.g., volume and pressure) to deliver one preset tidal volume, it is called:
    A. volume control.
    B. pressure control.
    C. dual control.
    D. servo control.

19. When a ventilator maintains a consistent volume waveform in the presence of changing compliance or resistance, the ventilator is used as a:
    A. flow controller.
    B. volume controller.
    C. time controller.
    D. A or B.

20. When a ventilator maintains a consistent volume waveform in the presence of changing compliance or resistance *and* measures the tidal volume and uses the signal to control the volume waveform, the ventilator is used as a:
    A. pressure controller.
    B. volume controller.
    C. time controller.
    D. dual controller.

Questions 21 to 23: Match the phase variables of a ventilator in Column I with the respective criteria in Column II. Use each answer ONCE.

Column I	Column II
21. Pressure triggered	A. Expiratory flow begins when a preset pressure is reached.
22. Pressure limited	B. Inspiration begins when a preset pressure is detected.
23. Pressure cycled	C. Pressure reaches a constant peak value before inspiration ends.

24. Positive end-expiratory pressure is a _____ variable.
    A. limit
    B. cycle
    C. trigger
    D. baseline

25. Refer to Figure 39-10 in the textbook. There are _____ control variables and the ventilator is able to control _____ variable at one time.
    A. one; one
    B. two; two
    C. three; one
    D. four; two

Questions 26 to 30: Match the terms in Column I with the respective definitions in Column II. Use each answer ONCE.

Column I   Column II

26. Mandatory breath   A. The ventilator delivers machine-triggered breaths, with spontaneous breaths allowed in between.
27. Continuous mandatory ventilation
                          B. The ventilator delivers intermittent (patient- or machine-triggered) mandatory breaths, with spontaneous breaths allowed in between.
28. Intermittent mandatory ventilation
                          C. Inspiration is ventilator triggered and/or machine cycled.
29. Synchronized intermittent mandatory ventilation
                          D. Every breath is mandatory.
                          E. The ventilator attempts to maintain a preset airway pressure waveform during inspiration.
30. Pressure control

31. In classifying the mode of ventilation, the *primary breath control* variables include all of the following *except*:
    A. volume.
    B. time.
    C. pressure.
    D. dual.

32. In classifying the mode of ventilation, the *breath sequences* include all of the following *except*:
    A. pressure control ventilation (PCV).
    B. continuous mandatory ventilation (CMV).
    C. intermittent mandatory ventilation (IMV).
    D. continuous spontaneous ventilation (CSV).

33. In addition to the breathing pattern, the ventilator mode classification scheme considers the:
    A. type of control strategy.
    B. specific control strategy.
    C. operational logic.
    D. all of the above.

34. A control circuit is the subsystem responsible for controlling the drive mechanism and/or the output control valve. The available control circuits include:
    A. mechanical.
    B. pneumatic, fluidic.
    C. electric, electronic
    D. all of the above.

35. Compressor, motor and linkage, and electric motor are some examples of the _____ mechanism of a ventilator.
    A. control
    B. drive
    C. output
    D. alarm

36. The output control valve is used to:
    A. control the pressure limit.
    B. regulate the flow of gas from the patient.
    C. regulate the flow of gas to the patient.
    D. measure the expired tidal volume.

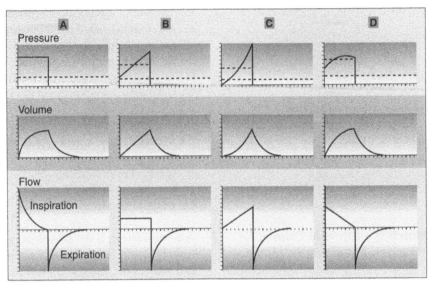

Typical pressure, volume, and flow waveforms during mechanical ventilation.

37. In the figure shown above, ascending flow pattern is seen under Column _____.
    A. A
    B. B
    C. C
    D. D

38. In addition to the rectangular (square) output waveform, the ventilator can produce _____ output waveforms.
    A. exponential
    B. ramp
    C. sinusoidal
    D. all of the above

39. The _____ alarm goes off when the rechargeable battery source is running low.
    A. control circuit
    B. input power
    C. output
    D. apnea

Questions 40 to 45: Match the types of output alarms in Column I with the clinical conditions in Column II. You may use any answer MORE THAN ONCE.

Column I

40. High pressure alarm

41. Low pressure alarm

42. Inspired gas temperature alarm

43. Low volume alarm

44. Failure to return to baseline pressure alarm

45. High minute volume alarm

Column II

A. Cuff leak
B. Patient increases spontaneous respiratory rate and volume
C. Exhalation manifold malfunction
D. Kinked endotracheal tube
E. Incorrect placement of temperature probe

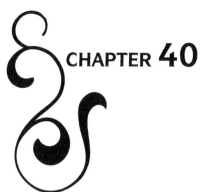

CHAPTER 40

Mechanical Ventilation

1. Mechanical ventilation is indicated in clinical conditions that may lead to:
   A. chronic ventilatory failure.
   B. impending respiratory alkalosis.
   C. hypoxemia.
   D. apnea.

2. Mr. Burns, a patient in the intensive unit, has been mechanically ventilated for three weeks. Sputum culture and chest radiograph confirm the presence of ventilator-associated pneumonia. This condition is most likely caused by:
   A. aspiration of oropharyngeal secretions.
   B. poor suctioning technique.
   C. use of inline suction device.
   D. incorrect use of antibiotics.

Questions 3 to 8. Match the types of complications of mechanical ventilation in Column I with the respective examples in Column II. Use each answer ONCE.

Column I

3. Airway complications

4. Mechanical complications

5. Pulmonary complications

6. Cardiovascular complications

7. Renal complications

8. Neurologic complications

Column II

A. Ventilator-induced lung injury
B. Laryngeal edema
C. Reduced urine output
D. Circuit disconnection
E. Increased intracranial pressure
F. Reduced venous return and cardiac output

9. Dr. Penn, a first-year resident, asks you to describe the strategy to minimize overdistention (volutrauma) during mechanical ventilation. You would suggest keeping the:
   A. peak airway pressure less than 50 cm H_2O.
   B. end-inspiratory plateau pressure less than 30 cm H_2O.
   C. positive end-expiratory pressure less than 10 cm H_2O.
   D. tidal volume less than 6 mL/kg.

10. Permissive hypercapnia is a lung protection strategy that allows a high _____ level during mechanical ventilation by using low _____.
    A. SpO_2; peak inspiratory pressure
    B. SpO_2; tidal volume
    C. $PaCO_2$; peak inspiratory pressure
    D. $PaCO_2$; tidal volume

11. Dr. Sanchez has ordered pressure support ventilation for her patient in the surgical intensive care unit. To benefit from this mode of ventilation, the patient must:
    A. be breathing spontaneously.
    B. have normal blood gases.
    C. have normal cardiac output.
    D. be using a pressure ventilator.

12. When pressure support ventilation is used alone, the _____ is determined by the level of pressure support.
    A. respiratory rate
    B. inspiratory flow
    C. tidal volume
    D. inspiratory time

13. When the ventilator switches from pressure control to volume control during a breath, it is called:
    A. SIMV mode.
    B. control mode.
    C. assist/control mode.
    D. dual mode.

14. Pressure-trigger or flow-trigger is initiated by the _____ immediately before a _____ tidal volume breath.
    A. ventilator; mechanical
    B. ventilator; spontaneous
    C. patient; mechanical
    D. patient; spontaneous

15. The compliance of Mr. Yarbrough, a patient being ventilated with volume-control ventilation, has been decreasing gradually over the past two days. On the patient's ventilator flow sheets, you would expect to see a corresponding _____ in _____.
    A. increase; lung volume
    B. increase; peak airway pressure
    C. decrease; lung volume
    D. decrease; peak airway pressure

16. Ms. Warren is being ventilated with pressure-control ventilation. Her physician asks you to increase the delivered mechanical tidal volume. You would:
    A. increase the peak inspiratory pressure.
    B. increase the peak flow.
    C. decrease the inspiratory time.
    D. decrease the level of auto-PEEP.

Questions 17 to 19: Match the patient conditions in Column I with the recommended tidal volume settings in Column II. Use each answer ONCE.

Column I   Column II

17. Normal lung function   A. 6 mL/Kg
                                  B. 8 to 10 mL/Kg
18. Obstructive lung disease   C. 10 to 12 mL/Kg

19. Respiratory distress
    syndrome

20. Positive end-expiratory pressure is used to provide _____ and correct _____.
    A. alveolar recruitment; dead space ventilation
    B. alveolar recruitment; intrapulmonary shunting
    C. normal tidal volume; dead space ventilation
    D. normal tidal volume; intrapulmonary shunting

21. When using a ventilator that does not compensate for circuit compliance, circuits with _____ compliance should be used in order to maintain the delivered _____.
    A. low; volume
    B. low; pressure
    C. high; volume
    D. high; pressure

22. A heat and moisture exchanger is used during mechanical ventilation to provide:
    A. air conditioning.
    B. positive end-expiratory pressure.
    C. filtering function.
    D. humidification.

23. Assessment of the symmetry of chest wall movement may be used to evaluate the presence of all of the following conditions *except*:
    A. main-stem intubation.
    B. tracheal obstruction.
    C. atelectasis.
    D. pneumothorax.

24. During your clinical rotation through the intensive care unit, you notice a therapist performing a maneuver using an end-expiratory pause of one second. This is done to:
    A. evaluate the presence of auto-PEEP.
    B. determine the plateau pressure.
    C. measure the I:E ratio.
    D. shorten the inspiratory time.

25. In reviewing the pressure-volume curve on the graphic display of a ventilator, you observe that the lower inflection point is 8 cm H_2O. Using this information, you would initially set the _____ and reevaluate the outcome.
    A. peak airway pressure at 38 cm H_2O
    B. plateau pressure at 38 cm H_2O
    C. PEEP at 8 cm H_2O
    D. CPAP at 8 cm H_2O

26. Point A in the figure shown on page 115 represents the _____, and the _____ plateau pressure during mechanical ventilation should be kept below this point.
    A. upper inflection point; peak airway
    B. upper inflection point; plateau airway
    C. lower inflection point; peak airway
    D. lower inflection point; plateau airway

27. _____ dyssynchrony is a condition in which the patient has difficulty initiating a mechanical breath.
    A. Flow
    B. Cycle
    C. Mode
    D. Trigger

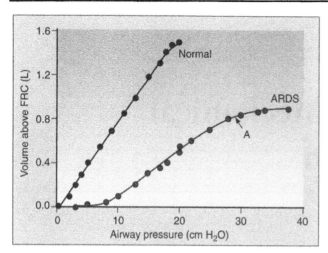

Pressure-volume curves for normal lungs and those of individuals with ARDS.

28. Dr. Manning asks you to evaluate his patient for weaning readiness. After measuring the weaning parameters, you would report that all of the following measurements indicated weaning readiness *except:*
    A. $V_D/V_T = 0.5$.
    B. $PaO_2 = 70$ on an F_1O_2 of 40%.
    C. rapid, shallow breathing index = 140.
    D. spontaneous tidal volume = 6 mL/kg.

29. T-piece, SIMV, and pressure support ventilation are useful tools during the _____ process of mechanical ventilation.
    A. oxygenation
    B. weaning
    C. ventilatory
    D. intubation

30. Three hours following the start of the weaning trial of a patient, you observe the following measurements: heart rate = 110/min; BP = 144/89 mm Hg; respiratory rate = 30/min; SpO_2 = 92%. Based on these observations, you would _____ the weaning trial and

    _____.
    A. terminate; place the patient back on mechanical ventilation
    B. terminate; place the patient on pressure support ventilation
    C. continue with; monitor the patient
    D. continue with; order stat blood gases and chest radiograph.

CHAPTER 41

Neonatal Mechanical Ventilation

Questions 1 to 5: You are called to the obstetric unit to assist in the delivery of a 32-week gestational age neonate. Following delivery, a small amount of meconium is noted in the mouth and nostrils.

1. While the nurse is drying and warming the neonate, _____ should be done to the neonate concurrently.
   A. suctioning of the oral and nasal cavities
   B. bag-mask ventilation
   C. positive-pressure ventilation
   D. intubation

2. The neonate remains apneic 30 seconds after birth and little spontaneous efforts are observed. Since there is no evidence of meconium below the vocal cords, you would provide tactile stimulation and _____ with a _____.
   A. positive-pressure ventilation; flow-inflating bag
   B. positive-pressure ventilation; self-inflating bag
   C. bag-mask ventilation; flow-inflating bag
   D. bag-mask ventilation; self-inflating bag

3. Effectiveness of ventilation to overcome the surfactant-deficient lungs can be done by observing the:
   A. appearance of cyanosis.
   B. rise of chest wall.
   C. pulse oximetry reading.
   D. heart rate.

4. In providing bag-mask ventilation to the neonate, you would keep the respiratory rate from _____ breaths per minute and inspiratory time from _____ seconds.
   A. 20 to 40; 0.4 to 0.5
   B. 20 to 40; 0.5 to 1
   C. 40 to 60; 0.4 to 0.5
   D. 40 to 60; 0.5 to 1

5. Five minutes after birth, the neonate remains apneic and the heart rate averages 90/min. The SpO$_2$ is in the mid-90s via bag-mask ventilation with oxygen. You would recommend:
   A. oxygen therapy via non-rebreathing mask.
   B. continue with bag-mask ventilation.
   C. intubation and positive-pressure ventilation.
   D. aerosol therapy with albuterol.

6. In infants with evidence of a large amount of meconium below the vocal cords, _____ must be done prior to initiation of positive-pressure ventilation.
   A. repeated endotracheal intubation and suctioning
   B. repeated nasotracheal suctioning
   C. bronchoscopy
   D. chest radiography and arterial blood gases

7. Indications for nasal continuous positive airway pressure include all of the following *except*:
   A. apnea.
   B. low spontaneous tidal volume.
   C. hypoxemia.
   D. tracheomalacia.

8. You are called to the high-risk nursery to intubate a neonate weighing 1500 g. You would select a(n) _____ endotracheal tube.
   A. cuffed, size 2.5
   B. cuffed, size 3
   C. uncuffed, size 2.5
   D. uncuffed, size 3

9. A neonate is being evaluated to rule out the presence of persistent pulmonary hypertension of the neonate (PPHN). The following SpO$_2$ readings are recorded: right digit SpO$_2$ = 92%; left digit SpO$_2$ = 91%. This information _____ confirm the diagnosis of PPHN and _____ should be done.
   A. does; cardiac ultrasound
   B. does; right radial and umbilical blood gases
   C. does not; cardiac ultrasound
   D. does not; right radial and umbilical blood gases

10. The tidal volume delivered by a neonatal positive-pressure ventilator is *least* likely to be affected by the _____ setting.
    A. oxygen concentration
    B. flow rate
    C. pressure gradient
    D. inspiratory time

Questions 11 to 13: A neonate is being mechanically ventilated with the following settings: peak inspiratory pressure (PIP) = 12 cm H₂O, positive end-expiratory pressure (PEEP) = 2 cm H₂O, F₁O₂ = 40%, respiratory rate = 20/min, flow = 8 L/min. On these settings, the SpO₂ = 89%.

11. Due to persistent hypoxemia, Dr. Leyham increased the PEEP level to 4 cm H_2O. Thirty minutes later, the SpO_2 reads 87%. This change in SpO_2 reading is the direct result of:
    A. decreased cardiac output.
    B. decreased tidal volume.
    C. increased dead space.
    D. increased shunting.

12. The answer in question #11 is due to the effect of:
    A. positive-pressure ventilation.
    B. reduced pressure gradient.
    C. reduced tidal volume.
    D. atelectasis.

13. To correct this problem, you would recommend:
    A. decreasing the PIP to 10 cm H_2O.
    B. decreasing the PEEP to 3 cm H_2O.
    C. increasing the PIP to 14 cm H_2O.
    D. increasing the PEEP to 5 cm H_2O.

14. The peak inspiratory pressure setting on a neonatal ventilator should be adjusted until a _____ of _____ is obtained.
    A. tidal volume; 5 to 7 mL/kg
    B. tidal volume; 7 to 10 mL/kg
    C. SpO_2; 90% to 95%
    D. SpO_2; 95% to 100%

15. Dr. King asks you to set up a neonatal ventilator at a rate of 25/min and use a mode of ventilation so that the neonate may breathe between these 25 breaths. You would select the _____ mode.
    A. pressure control (PC)
    B. synchronized intermittent mandatory ventilation (SIMV)
    C. continuous mandatory ventilation (CMV)
    D. continuous positive airway pressure (CPAP)

16. Given: respiratory rate = 40/min, inspiratory time = 0.5 sec. The inspiratory:expiratory (I:E) ratio is:
    A. 1:1.
    B. 1:1.5.
    C. 1:2.
    D. 1:2.5.

17. Air trapping and auto-PEEP are conditions commonly associated with:
    A. inadequate inspiratory time.
    B. inadequate expiratory time.
    C. prolonged expiratory time.
    D. I:E ratio of 1:3.

18. Dr. Wentworth asks you to initiate PEEP on a neonate in order to improve the oxygenation status. You would start PEEP at _____ and evaluate the neonate.
    A. 1 to 3 cm H_2O
    B. 3 to 5 cm H_2O
    C. 5 to 7 cm H_2O
    D. 7 to 9 cm H_2O

19. Pneumonia, tracheal damage, reduced cerebral blood flow, and bronchopulmonary dysplasia are some hazards and complications associated with _____ in the neonate.
    A. prolonged intubation
    B. 100% oxygen therapy
    C. continuous positive airway pressure
    D. mechanical ventilation

20. Weaning in the SIMV mode is done by decreasing the _____ rate gradually. This strategy causes an increase of the neonate's _____.
    A. spontaneous; compliance
    B. spontaneous; work of breathing
    C. mandatory; compliance
    D. mandatory; work of breathing

21. Baby Johnson is being weaned from mechanical ventilation. The most recent parameters on the ventilator are as follows: rate = 16/min, PIP = 14 cm H_2O, PEEP = 3 cm H_2O, F₁O₂ = 30%. Blood gases and vital signs are normal. You would recommend to the physician that:
    A. the PIP should be decreased to 12 cm H_2O.
    B. the rate be decreased to 14/min.
    C. Baby Johnson be extubated.
    D. the PEEP be discontinued.

Questions 22 to 25: Match the types of high-frequency ventilation in Column I with the respective characteristics in Column II. Use each answer ONCE.

Column I

Column II

22. High-frequency positive-pressure ventilation (HFPPV)

23. High-frequency jet ventilation (HFJV)

24. High-frequency flow interrupter ventilation (HFFIV)

25. High-frequency oscillatory ventilation (HFPPV)

A. Provides inspiratory flow by airway vibrations; rates = 400 to 2400/min; inspiration and exhalation are active.

B. Provides inspiratory flow in short bursts; rates = 2 to 22 Hz (120 to 1320/min); inspiration and exhalation are active.

C. Provides small tidal volume by conventional positive-pressure ventilation at rate >150/min; exhalation is passive.

D. Provides tidal volume that is equal to or less than dead space volume; rates = 150 to 600/min; exhalation is passive.

26. *Spike formation, helical diffusion, Taylor dispersion, pendelluft ventilation,* and *molecular diffusion* are terms associated with the _____ theories during high-frequency ventilation.
    A. gas transport
    B. oxygenation
    C. ventilation
    D. gas diffusion

27. Use of high-frequency ventilation should be considered in all of the following patient conditions *except:*
    A. severe hyaline membrane disease with PIP > 30 cm H_2O.
    B. severe meconium aspiration syndrome and persistent pulmonary hypertension refractory to ventilatory support with PIP > 35 cm H_2O.
    C. air leak syndrome.
    D. ventilator-associated pneumonia.

Questions 28 to 30: Match the types of high-frequency ventilators in Column I with the respective characteristics in Column II. Use each answer ONCE.

Column I

Column II

28. Infant Star 950

29. Bunnell Life Pulse Jet Ventilator

30. SensorMedics 3100A

A. Relies on conventional ventilator to provide continuous gas flow and low rate IMV; uses a special triple lumen (Hi-Lo Jet) endotracheal tube during HFJV.

B. Oscillatory pressure amplitude and mean airway pressure are two primary controls; does not require a special endotracheal tube.

C. Capable of delivering HFV by itself or as an adjunct to IMV; target patient size = 600 to 2250 g.

31. A(n) _____ jet servo pressure on the Bunnell Life Pulse ventilator reflects an improvement of the neonates' _____ .
    A. increasing; compliance
    B. increasing; compliance and resistance
    C. decreasing; compliance
    D. decreasing; compliance and resistance

32. On the SensorMedics 3100A ventilator, the mean airway pressure control determines the neonate's:
    A. tidal volume.
    B. respiratory rate.
    C. end-expiratory pressure.
    D. end-expiratory lung volume.

33. In HFV, the mean airway pressure and end-expiratory lung volume are determined by the _____ setting.
    A. tidal volume
    B. PEEP
    C. amplitude
    D. peak inspiratory pressure

34. In HFOV, ventilation is determined by all of the following controls *except:*
    A. mean airway pressure.
    B. percent inspiratory time.
    C. respiratory rate.
    D. amplitude.

35. In comparing HFOV with HFJV, higher _____ are required to maintain oxygenation with _____.
    A. mean airway pressures; HFOV
    B. mean airway pressures; HFJV
    C. amplitude; HFOV
    D. amplitude; HFJV

36. Complications associated with HFV include all of the following *except*:
    A. pulmonary overdistention.
    B. atelectasis.
    C. hypertension.
    D. hyperventilation.

Questions 37 to 38: You are getting ready to suction an orally intubated neonate via an inline suction catheter.

37. In order to avoid airway trauma, you would insert the suction catheter to a length of no more than _____ cm plus the distance from the neonate's _____ to the distal end of the inline catheter fully withdrawn.
    A. 0.2; lips
    B. 0.2; nares
    C. 0.5; lips
    D. 0.5; nares

38. You would use a vacuum pressure between _____ mm Hg to suction this neonate.
    A. 10 to 40
    B. 40 to 70
    C. 70 to 100
    D. 100 to 130

39. Baby Homer has a diagnosis of respiratory distress syndrome. During physical assessment, you would expect to see all of the following signs *except*:
    A. intercostal and sternal retraction.
    B. nasal flaring.
    C. tachypnea.
    D. inspiratory wheezing.

40. _____ is a synthetic surfactant administered _____.
    A. Survanta; by aerosol nebulizer
    B. Exosurf; endotracheally
    C. Curosurf; by aerosol nebulizer
    D. Infrasurf; endotracheally

41. Nitric oxide is a _____ used to treat _____ in neonates.
    A. vasoconstrictor; pulmonary edema
    B. bronchodilator; atelectasis
    C. vasodilator; pulmonary hypertension
    D. analgesic; ventilatory failure

42. Extracorporeal life support is done to improve _____ and reduce ventilating _____ in selected full-term neonates.
    A. ventilation; time
    B. ventilation; pressure
    C. oxygenation; time
    D. oxygenation; pressure

CHAPTER 42

Mechanical Ventilation in Alternate Care Sites

1. Alternate site mechanical ventilation is done to reduce costs of _____ medical care and to improve the quality of life for _____.
   A. short-term; family members
   B. short-term; ventilator-assisted individuals
   C. long-term; family members
   D. long-term; ventilator-assisted individuals

Questions 2 to 5: Match the settings where patients receive medical care in Column I with the type of facilities in Column II. You may use any answer MORE THAN ONCE.

Column I   Column II

2. Home   A. Acute care
                                  B. Intermediate care
3. Rehabilitation hospital   C. Long-term care

4. Intensive care unit

5. Assisted-living facility

6. Patients with _____ are most likely to be weaned from alternate site mechanical ventilation within one to three years.
   A. cervical trauma
   B. neuromuscular disease
   C. parenchymal lung disease
   D. amyotrophic lateral sclerosis

7. In skilled nursing facilities (SNFs), care of the patients receiving mechanical ventilation has been shifted from respiratory therapists to nurses because of changes in:
   A. professional qualification.
   B. reimbursement policy.
   C. patient demographics.
   D. technology.

8. Under the _____ reimbursement guidelines, hospitals began to place long-term mechanically ventilated patients outside the acute care setting.
   A. diagnosis-related group (DRG)
   B. prospective payment system (PPS)
   C. Medicare
   D. Medicaid

9. Settings that are available to ventilator-assisted individuals include all of the following *except*:
   A. home.
   B. hotel.
   C. SNF.
   D. assisted living in a group home.

10. In choosing the best site for a ventilator-assisted individual, _____ should *not* be the primary consideration.
    A. physician's preference
    B. patient's preference
    C. insurance coverage
    D. patient's medical needs

11. The type of ventilator selected for a ventilator-assisted individual should have all of the following features *except*:
    A. meeting the patient's ventilatory needs.
    B. easy to operate safely.
    C. functioning in a home setting without excessive accessories.
    D. identical to the ventilator in the hospital.

12. Most successful home care arrangements rely on _____ for routine care and _____ for regular respite.
    A. family members; equipment technicians
    B. family members; health care professionals
    C. equipment technicians; family members
    D. health care professionals; family members

13. Caring for a ventilator-assisted individual at home and around-the-clock can be a(n) _____ situation.
    A. busy
    B. happy
    C. stressful
    D. impossible

14. _____ can be the most important factors in considering which ventilator to use at home.
    A. Cost and reimbursement
    B. Location and transportation
    C. Electrical outlets and fire escape
    D. Experience and age of the care providers

15. _____ is the practice of billing a patient directly for any amount that exceeds the insurance payment.
    A. Medicare copayment
    B. Deductibles
    C. Medicare Part B
    D. Balanced billing

16. The older, first-generation, portable ventilators used in long-term care facilities are *least* likely to offer:
    A. continuous mandatory ventilation.
    B. pressure support ventilation.
    C. intermittent mandatory ventilation.
    D. positive end-expiratory pressure.

17. Bilevel positive airway pressure is a form of _____ positive-pressure ventilation and it _____ approved by the U.S. Food and Drug Administration to provide total ventilatory support.
    A. invasive; is not
    B. invasive; is
    C. noninvasive; is not
    D. noninvasive; is

18. One of the advantages of negative pressure ventilator is that it can provide ventilation without a(n):
    A. power source.
    B. artificial airway.
    C. physician's order.
    D. alarm.

Questions 19 to 21: Match the hazards and complications of mechanical ventilation in an alternate site in Column I with the respective examples in Column II. Use each answer ONCE.

Column I	Column II
19. Medical factors	A. Depression, anxiety, stress
20. Equipment-related factors	B. Ventilator malfunction, inadvertant changes in ventilator settings
21. Psychosocial factors	C. Hypoxemia, respiratory acid-base abnormalities, barotrauma

22. The ventilator circuit used in an alternate site should have all of the following characteristics *except:*
    A. proper length to suit the patient's needs.
    B. low noise level.
    C. high compliance.
    D. adequate humidity.

23. You are asked to provide instructions to the caretakers of Mr. Lange, a ventilator-dependent patient who is being sent home with a mechanical ventilator. For the parameters that should be monitored regularly, you would include:
    A. vital signs.
    B. ventilator settings.
    C. alarms.
    D. all of the above.

24. If at all possible, the respiratory therapist should use the _____ ventilator for the transport of a ventilator-dependent patient between home and destination.
    A. patient's
    B. long-term care facility's
    C. acute care facility's
    D. manual

25. Prior to discharge from the hospital and beginning using a ventilator at home, the patient must have:
    A. a positive attitude.
    B. involved and capable family members.
    C. workable financial resources.
    D. all of the above.

CHAPTER 43 Noninvasive Ventilation and Continuous Positive Airway Pressure

1. *Noninvasive ventilation* may be defined as use of mechanical ventilation:
   A. for a period no longer than one day.
   B. for a period no longer than one week.
   C. at home.
   D. without an endotracheal or tracheostomy tube.

2. Clinical applications or benefits of noninvasive positive pressure ventilation in an *acute* care setting includes all of the following *except:*
   A. lower incidence of ventilator-associated pneumonia.
   B. weaning patients with COPD from mechanical ventilation.
   C. reducing staff time in the care of patients with COPD.
   D. lower intubation rate.

Questions 3 to 4: Dr. Singer asks you to evaluate his patient for the feasibility of noninvasive positive-pressure ventilation (NPPV). The patient, Mr. Jones, has a primary diagnosis of COPD and is being treated for acute respiratory distress in the emergency department.

3. In evaluation Mr. Jones, all of the following would meet the *selection* criteria for use of NPPV *except:*
   A. presence of upper airway obstruction.
   B. reversibility of patient's condition.
   C. presence of moderate to severe dyspnea.
   D. presence of acute hypercapnia.

4. In evaluation Mr. Jones, all of the following would meet the *exclusion* criteria for use of NPPV *except:*
   A. presence of impaired neurological state.
   B. presence of acute respiratory acidosis.
   C. recent facial trauma.
   D. unable to handle secretions.

5. In addition to patients with COPD, *chronic* application of NPPV may include patients with:
   A. restrictive lung disease.
   B. nocturnal hypoventilation.
   C. severe neuromuscular disease.
   D. all of the above.

6. Nasal mask, oronasal mask, full face mask, and nasal pillows are _____ used in NPPV.
   A. adapters
   B. interfaces
   C. noninvasive airways
   D. ventilation masks

7. In comparison to a nasal mask used during NPPV, an oronasal mask offers:
   A. easier secretion clearance.
   B. less risk of aspiration.
   C. greater effectiveness for dyspneic patients.
   D. decreased claustrophobia.

8. Increased dead space, significant air leak, and increased aspiration risk are some disadvantages of a(n):
   A. oronasal mask.
   B. nasal pillow.
   C. nasal mask.
   D. all of the above.

9. In selecting and fitting the interface on a new patient, a common mistake is choosing an interface that is too _____ or fitting the headgear too _____.
   A. large; loosely
   B. large; tightly
   C. small; loosely
   D. small; tightly

10. When a NPPV ventilator is used, pressure support is provided by the:
    A. inspiratory positive airway pressure (IPAP).
    B. expiratory positive airway pressure (EPAP).
    C. difference between IPAP and EPAP.
    D. positive end-expiratory pressure.

11. In addition to ventilation support, a typical NPPV ventilator is capable of providing:
    A. supplemental oxygen.
    B. inline nebulizer therapy.
    C. humidity.
    D. all of the above.

12. Based on Figure 43-6 of the textbook, the algorithm for NPPV to treat acute respiratory failure, the initial step prior to implementation of NPPV is to:
    A. evaluate the inclusion and exclusion criteria.
    B. select a proper interface.
    C. titrate the initial IPAP and EPAP levels.
    D. obtain an arterial blood gas sample.

13. Mr. Hightower, a patient with COPD, has been using NPPV for several hours. Which of the following changes is considered a positive *physiologic* response to NPPV?
    A. Decrease in sensation of dyspnea.
    B. Decrease in spontaneous respiratory rate.
    C. Improvement in SpO_2 measurements.
    D. Improvement in neurological status.

14. Negative pressure ventilators are _____ for patients with obstructive sleep apnea because these ventilators tend to _____.
    A. indicated; relieve upper airway obstruction
    B. indicated; relieve intrapulmonary shunting
    C. contraindicated; produce oxygen toxicity
    D. contraindicated; produce upper airway obstruction

15. Mask CPAP (continuous positive airway pressure) is indicated for patients with acute _____ pulmonary edema because the increase in intrathoracic pressure causes a(n) _____ in preload and afterload.
    A. cardiogenic; increase
    B. cardiogenic; decrease
    C. noncardiogenic; increase
    D. noncardiogenic; decrease

16. Dr. Lambert asks you to start CPAP for her patient in the coronary intensive care unit. You would set the initial CPAP level from _____ cm H_2O and reassess the patient for adjustments.
    A. 2 to 5
    B. 5 to 8
    C. 8 to 12
    D. 12 to 16

17. Chronic conditions such as _____ may benefit from CPAP.
    A. obstructive sleep apnea
    B. central sleep apnea
    C. combined apnea
    D. upper airway edema

18. The ramp/delay feature during nocturnal CPAP therapy is used to help a patient to:
    A. avoid excessive noise from machine.
    B. relieve upper airway obstruction.
    C. breathe better.
    D. fall asleep.

19. Common complaints from CPAP users include all of the following *except*:
    A. nasal congestion.
    B. dryness in mouth.
    C. epistaxis (nosebleed).
    D. chest pain.

20. With a bilevel positive airway pressure system, the _____ level is adjusted to eliminate apneas, hypopneas, and snoring.
    A. IPAP
    B. EPAP
    C. CPAP
    D. PEEP

21. The auto-positive airway pressure (APAP) device is ideal for patients who have frequent, changing _____ requirements.
    A. body position
    B. pressure
    C. volume
    D. oxygenation

CHAPTER 44

Nonconventional Respiratory Therapeutics

1. Nitric oxide:
   A. does not diffuse across cell membranes to adjacent cells.
   B. is a pulmonary vasodilator when inhaled.
   C. is absent in exhaled gas.
   D. can be used as a bronchodilator.

2. Nitric oxide:
   A. reduces pulmonary vascular resistance.
   B. reduces pulmonary blood flow.
   C. increases dead space ventilation.
   D. increases intrapulmonary shunting.

3. Inhaled nitric oxide (NO) differs from intravenous vasodilators in that NO has minimal _____ effect.
   A. pulmonary vasodilation
   B. pulmonary vasoconstriction
   C. systemic vasodilation
   D. systemic vasoconstriction

4. Inhaled NO has been used successfully in the treatment and support of _____ with _____.
   A. adults; systemic hypertension
   B. adults; pulmonary hypertension
   C. neonates; systemic hypertension
   D. neonates; pulmonary hypertension

5. The usual starting concentration of inhaled NO is:
   A. 20 parts per million.
   B. 80 parts per million.
   C. 20 parts per billion.
   D. 80 parts per billion.

6. _____ is produced when NO is exposed to oxygen and it may produce toxic effects on the lungs such as _____.
   A. Nitrogen dioxide (NO_2); airway reactivity and parenchymal lung injury
   B. Nitrogen dioxide (NO_2); oxygen toxicity and atelectasis
   C. Nitrous oxide (N_2O); airway reactivity and parenchymal lung injury
   D. Nitrous oxide (N_2O); oxygen toxicity and atelectasis

7. In some patients with severe left ventricular dysfunction, inhaled NO (at doses from 40 to 80 ppm):
   A. increases the pulmonary vascular resistance.
   B. increases the pulmonary wedge pressure.
   C. decreases the pulmonary blood flow to left ventricle.
   D. decreases the left ventricular filling pressure and volume.

8. To prevent the harmful effects of rebound during withdrawal of inhaled NO:
   A. use the lowest effective dose (5 ppm or less).
   B. continue NO until patient's clinical status has improved.
   C. set the NO dose at 20 ppm for a short time before discontinuance.
   D. discontinue oxygen to prevent formation of NO_2.

9. Inhaled nitric oxide (NO) delivery system can be used with:
   A. adult and neonatal ventilators.
   B. anesthesia machines.
   C. spontaneously breathing patients.
   D. all of the above.

10. Heliox _____ support life and it requires _____ oxygen in the gas mixture.
    A. does; no
    B. does; less than 20%
    C. does not; at least 20%
    D. does not; 100%

Questions 11 to 13: Mr. Busbee, a patient in the recovery room following surgery, has developed mild stridor soon after extubation. His physician orders Heliox therapy via simple mask to relieve hypoxemia.

11. A member of Mr. Busbee's family asks you about the purpose of Heliox therapy. In your discussion, you would explain that Heliox is used to:
    A. reduce peak flow.
    B. reduce air flow resistance.
    C. increase $PaCO_2$.
    D. increase peak airway pressure.

12. If you use an oxygen flow meter to deliver 5 L/min of Heliox to Mr. Busbee, what is the actual flow rate?
    A. 9 L/min
    B. 11 L/min
    C. 15 L/min
    D. Insufficient information to determine answer

13. To assess the clinical benefits of Heliox, you would look for all of the following signs *except:*
    A. decreased work of breathing.
    B. decreased stridor.
    C. increased pulsus paradoxus.
    D. increased quality of breath sounds.

14. _____ is the technique of injecting fresh gas into the central airway to improve alveolar ventilation and reduce work of breathing.
    A. Tracheal gas exsufflation
    B. Tracheal gas insufflation
    C. Prone positioning
    D. Heliox therapy

15. Prone positioning is beneficial to patients with _____ but contraindicated in those with _____.
    A. pulmonary edema; tension pneumothorax
    B. pulmonary edema; spinal cord injury
    C. ARDS; tension pneumothorax
    D. ARDS; spinal cord injury

16. The beneficial effects of prone positioning are the result of:
    A. increased intrapulmonary shunting.
    B. increased dead space ventilation.
    C. decreased work of breathing.
    D. improved ventilation/perfusion relationship.

17. CPAP, PEEP, and sigh breaths play an important role in _____ because of their ability to sustain inflation at _____.
    A. prone positioning; low lung volumes
    B. liquid ventilation; low lung volumes
    C. recruitment maneuver; high airway pressure
    D. Heliox therapy; high airway pressure

CHAPTER 45

Principles of Disease Management

1. In 1900, _____ diseases were common; whereas in 2000, chronic _____ diseases are prevalent.
   A. infectious; lifestyle
   B. infectious; cardiopulmonary
   C. lifestyle; infectious
   D. cardiopulmonary; infectious

2. Among the behavior causes of death in the United States, _____ is the leading cause of total deaths.
   A. alcohol use
   B. suicide
   C. inappropriate diet
   D. tobacco use

3. A patient asks you to describe the goals of disease management. In your description, you would include all of the following *except:*
   A. optimize profit for health care organizations.
   B. contain health care cost paid by health care consumers.
   C. expand the scope of practice for health care professionals.
   D. provide quality care to health care consumers.

4. _____ management is a clinical management process of care that spans the continuum of care from primary prevention to ongoing long-term health maintenance for patients with chronic health conditions or diagnoses.
   A. Case
   B. Component
   C. Demand
   D. Disease

5. _____ management deals with patients with multiple diseases; places its emphasis on the treatment of sickness; caregivers include generalists and nurses.
   A. Component
   B. Case
   C. Disease
   D. Demand

6. _____ management deals with patients with a single disease; places its emphasis on the prevention and education of the patient; caregivers include specialists and a multidisciplinary team of health care providers.
   A. Case
   B. Disease
   C. Component
   D. Demand

7. Emphasis of primary and secondary disease prevention and use of clinical guidelines and practice protocols are some factors associated with _____ management.
   A. disease
   B. demand
   C. component
   D. case

8. Health care value is enhanced when the _____ of care is high and the _____ is low.
   A. quantity; total cost
   B. quantity; staffing
   C. quality; total cost
   D. quality; staffing

9. In assessing health care value, the number of mortalities, morbidities, and complications may be measured to document the quality of _____ outcomes.
   A. service
   B. clinical
   C. economic
   D. humanistic

Questions 10 to 14: Match the cost drivers of disease in Column I with the respective descriptions or examples in Column II. Use each answer ONCE.

Column I

10. Compliance

11. Prevention

12. Rapid resolution

13. Acute flare-ups

14. The 80-20 Rule

Column II

A. Identifying the trigger and using treatments properly to avoid hospitalization.

B. Following treatment protocols to recover from illness completely.

C. Targeting the at-risk patient population for the prevention and treatment of illness.

D. Practicing safe sex to reduce the likelihood of acquiring sexually transmitted diseases.

E. Seeking medical attention as soon as feasible to avoid sustained or more serious illness.

15. In a patient education and compliance program for chronic disease management, _____ involvement and _____ of the disease are the key to success.
A. patient; self-management
B. patient; insurance coverage
C. family member; self-management
D. family member; insurance coverage

16. Asthma, congestive heart failure, and chronic obstructive pulmonary disease are illnesses most suited for disease management intervention because of which of the following characteristics?
   I. Low incidence of preventable complications
   II. Chronic nature of illnesses
   III. A small patient population
   IV. Measurable outcomes
A. I, II, and III only
B. I and III only
C. II and IV only
D. II, III, and IV only

17. You are appointed to take part in the development of a disease management program for COPD. The initial step would be to:
A. create a system for process and outcome measurement and reporting.
B. evaluate the benefits, harms, and costs.
C. generate specific clinical and economic questions and search the literature.
D. formulate a definition of COPD, its scope and its impact over time using a team of health care providers.

18. One of the obstacles to implementing disease management is the lack of useful and complete patient data for a given disease. This obstacle may be resolved by a(n):
A. computerized patient information system.
B. signed informed consent by each patient with COPD.
C. increase in funding for the disease management program.
D. enforcement of patient rights and responsibilities.

CHAPTER 46

Asthma

1. Asthma mortality is largely _____ and the death rates from this lung disease are highest in people _____ than 35 years of age.
   A. preventable; older
   B. preventable; younger
   C. not preventable; older
   D. not preventable; younger

Questions 2 to 3: Mr. Benson, a 55-year-old patient with chronic asthma in the pulmonary unit, asks you to tell him about the causes of wheezing and changes in the lungs with asthma.

2. You would tell Mr. Benson that wheezing is due to:
   A. excessive secretions in the lungs.
   B. dried secretions in the lungs.
   C. narrowing of the large airways.
   D. narrowing of the large or small airways.

3. You would also tell him that asthma is a result of all of the following changes in the lung parenchyma and airways *except*:
   A. hyperventilation.
   B. airway inflammation.
   C. easy and frequent constriction of airways.
   D. air flow obstruction.

4. Mast cells, eosinophils, macrophages, epithelial cells, and T lymphocytes are mediators that play an important role in the mechanism of airway _____ in asthma.
   A. obstruction
   B. inflammation
   C. hyperresponsiveness
   D. remodeling

5. In asthma, airway hyperresponsiveness may be due to:
   A. viral infection.
   B. indoor or outdoor pollution.
   C. exercise.
   D. all of the above.

6. Beta-agonists are best suited to reverse _____.
   A. bronchospasm
   B. edema
   C. inflammation
   D. hyperresponsiveness

7. Animal dander, mold, dust mites, and pollen are examples of _____ that may trigger an asthma response.
   A. food additives
   B. microbes
   C. allergens
   D. pollution

8. Nitric oxide, carbon monoxide, sulfur dioxide, and formaldehydes are examples of _____ that may trigger an asthma response.
   A. pollution
   B. allergens
   C. food additives
   D. microbes

9. Ms. Davidson, a 22-year-old college tennis team member, is being tested for exercise-induced asthma. The changes in selected pulmonary function parameters are shown below. Which parameters would be indicative of exercise-induced asthma?
   I. After-exercise FEV_1 is 12% lower than before-exercise FEV_1.
   II. After-exercise tidal volume is 15% lower than before-exercise tidal volume.
   III. After-exercise peak flow is 13% lower than before-exercise peak flow.
   A. I and II
   B. I and III
   C. II and III
   D. I, II, and III

Questions 10 and 11: *Mr. Caine, a patient with asthma, is in the emergency department being treated for asthma. In his recent history, he reports symptoms of coughing and wheezing almost every day and severe shortness of breath at least two times per week. Furthermore, he performs at the "yellow zone" on his peak flow meter.*

10. Based on this information, Mr. Caine may be classified as having _____ asthma.
    A. mild intermittent
    B. mild persistent
    C. moderate persistent
    D. severe persistent

11. Following three bronchodilator treatments in the emergency department, Mr. Caine's condition worsens. Arterial blood gases reveal hypercapnia and severe hypoxemia in spite of 90%+ inspired oxygen via non-rebreathing mask. His condition may be called:
    A. respiratory failure.
    B. combined acidosis.
    C. status asthmaticus.
    D. oxygenation failure.

Questions 12 and 13: *Mr. Goodman, a patient newly diagnosed with asthma, is getting ready to be discharged from the hospital. His physician, Dr. Panola, asks you to perform a test for the reversibility of airflow obstruction.*

12. You would measure the patient's _____ before and after giving _____ therapy.
    A. lung volumes; IPPB
    B. lung volumes; bronchodilator
    C. flow rates; IPPB
    D. flow rates; bronchodilator

13. In order to document airflow reversibility, the _____ measured after the therapy must be 12% to 15% _____ than that measured before the therapy.
    A. lung volumes; higher
    B. lung volumes; lower
    C. flow rates; higher
    D. flow rates; lower

14. Proper instruction and active coaching are very important steps to accomplish before measuring a patient's _____ because this measurement is extremely effort-dependent.
    A. peak flow
    B. vital capacity
    C. tidal volume
    D. total lung capacity

Questions 15 to 19: *Match the types of long-term controller medications for asthma in Column I with the respective generic (brand) names. Use each answer ONCE.*

Column I

15. Corticosteroids (MDI)

16. Nonsteroidal antiinflammatories

17. Long-acting beta-agonists

18. Methylxanthines (oral)

19. Leukotriene modifiers (oral)

Column II

A. Theophylline (Slo-bid, Theo-24, Theo-Dur)
B. Fluticasone (Flovent), triamcinolone (Azmacort), beclomethasone (Beclovent, Vanceril)
C. Zafirlukast (Accolate), montelukast (Singulair)
D. Salmeterol (Serevent)
E. Cromolyn sodium (Intal), nedocromil (Tilade)

20. Salmeterol is a _____ beta-2 agonist and it _____ be used as a quick-relief medication in status asthmaticus.
    A. short-acting; should
    B. short-acting; should not
    C. long-acting; should
    D. long-acting; should not

21. Theophylline acts as a nonselective _____ and its current therapeutic serum range is _____ mg/L to minimize potential toxic effects.
    A. leukotriene modifier; 5 to 15
    B. leukotriene modifier; 15 to 20
    C. phosphodiesterase inhibitor; 5 to 15
    D. phosphodiesterase inhibitor; 15 to 20

Questions 22 to 24: *Match the types of quick-relief medications for asthma in Column I with the respective generic (brand) names in Column II. Use each answer ONCE.*

Column I

22. Short-acting beta-agonists

23. Anticholinergics

24. Methylxanthines (intravenous)

Column II

A. Terbutaline (Brethine, Brethaire, Bricanyl), albuterol (Xopenex, Proven-til, Ventolin), bitolterol (Tornalate)
B. Aminophylline
C. Ipratropium bromide (Atrovent)

25. With a small-volume nebulizer, the volume of medication that is deposited in the lower respiratory tract is estimated to be about:
    A. 10%.
    B. 30%.
    C. 50%.
    D. 70%.

26. A spacer is used in conjunction with a _____ and its function is to increase the _____ dose.
    A. small-volume nebulizer; effective
    B. small-volume nebulizer; delivered
    C. metered-dose inhaler; effective
    D. metered-dose inhaler; delivered

27. Heliox facilitates oxygen delivery to the lungs because of its:
    A. high density.
    B. low density.
    C. high diffusion rate.
    D. low diffusion rate.

28. Magnesium sulfate is beneficial in the management of _____ and its mode of action is _____ of acetylcholine and histamine release.
    A. chronic asthma; inhibition
    B. chronic asthma; synthesis
    C. status asthmaticus; inhibition
    D. status asthmaticus; synthesis

29. For patients with asthma, mechanical ventilation may be indicated in all of the following conditions *except:*
    A. decrease of absent breath sounds.
    B. hypocapnia.
    C. refractory hypoxemia.
    D. mental status deterioration.

30. During mechanical ventilation of patients with asthma, overdistention of the lungs may be avoided by using a tidal volume in the _____ range and keeping the _____ pressure below 35 cm H_2O.
    A. 5 to 8 mL/kg; plateau
    B. 5 to 8 mL/kg; peak
    C. 8 to 12 mL/kg; plateau
    D. 8 to 12 mL/kg; peak

31. Auto-PEEP is a sign of _____ and its effect on patient triggering may be minimized by applying _____.
    A. intrapulmonary shunting; pressure support
    B. intrapulmonary shunting; PEEP
    C. air trapping; pressure support
    D. air trapping; PEEP

32. NAEPP is a(n) _____ primarily for patients with asthma.
    A. support group
    B. educational program
    C. treatment facility
    D. government funding program

CHAPTER 47

Chronic Obstructive Pulmonary Disease

1. Chronic obstructive pulmonary disease includes all of the following conditions *except:*
   A. cystic fibrosis.
   B. chronic bronchitis.
   C. asthmatic bronchitis.
   D. emphysema.

Questions 2 to 4: Match the type of COPD in Column I with the respective descriptions and characteristics in Column II. Use each answer ONCE.

Column I   Column II

2. Chronic   A. Cough, dyspnea, and wheezing; lim-
   bronchitis   ited improvement with broncho-
                     dilators and corticosteroids
3. Asthmatic   B. Presence of cough and sputum pro-
   bronchitis   duction for three or more months in
                     two successive years; normal chest
4. Emphysema   radiograph and lung diffusion
                 C. Damage to the lung parenchyma; air
                    trapping, hyperinflation, and irre-
                    versible airflow limitations

5. Mr. King, a 75-year-old patient with COPD, has an FEV_1 of 45% of predicted normal. This is considered:
   A. normal lung function for age.
   B. mild (stage 1) COPD.
   C. moderate (stage 2) COPD.
   D. severe (stage 3) COPD.

6. In patients with _____, the airways typically show hyperplasia of surface mucous cells, enlargement of submucosal glands, excessive mucus, loss of cilia, and ciliary dyskinesia.
   A. emphysema
   B. respiratory distress syndrome
   C. asthmatic bronchitis
   D. chronic bronchitis

7. The major etiologies of COPD include all of the following causes *except:*
   A. alpha 1-antitrypsin deficiency.
   B. environmental pollution.
   C. oxygen toxicity.
   D. smoking.

Questions 8 to 14: Match the pathophysiologic changes of COPD in Column I with the correct statements in Column II. You may use any answer MORE THAN ONCE.

Column I   Column II

8. Decreased airflow resistance   A. This **is** a
                                      characteristic
9. Increased dyspnea   of COPD.
                                   B. This **is not** a
10. Increased peak flow   characteristic
                                      of COPD.
11. Hyperinflation of lungs

12. Increase in dead space ventilation

13. Increased intrapulmonary shunting

14. Shift of volume/pressure (compliance) curve upward and to the left

15. The most important element of the outpatient care of all patients with COPD is:
    A. vaccinations.
    B. bronchodilator therapy.
    C. smoking cessation.
    D. oxygen therapy.

16. For COPD patients, selection and prescription of drugs should use the following sequence (starting with first line drugs):
    I. Methylxanthines
    II. ß-agonists
    III. Anticholinergics
    IV. Steroids
    A. I, II, IV, III
    B. II, III, I, IV
    C. III, II, I, IV
    D. IV, II, III, I

17. Patients with COPD tend to have increased _____ muscle tone and decreased response to _____ drugs supplied to the airways.
    A. cholinergic; adrenergic
    B. cholinergic; steroidal
    C. adrenergic; cholinergic
    D. adrenergic; steroidal

18. In general, long-lasting ß-agonists have _____ onset and they _____ be used for rescue therapy.
    A. fast; should
    B. fast; are sometimes
    C. slow; are sometimes
    D. slow; should not

19. Methylxanthines (e.g., theophylline) are used as third-line drugs in the management of COPD because they have a _____ and the dosage is titrated to reach a serum concentration of _____ mg/dL.
    A. narrow therapeutic index; 5 to 15
    B. narrow therapeutic index; 10 to 20
    C. wide range of serious side effects; 5 to 15
    D. wide range of serious side effects; 10 to 20

20. Osteoporosis, diabetes, fluid retention, hypertension, and immunosuppression with risk of infection are some side effects of long-term _____ therapy.
    A. bronchodilator
    B. corticosteroid
    C. intravenous drug
    D. smoking cessation

Questions 21 to 23: Mr. Crowne, a patient with an admitting diagnosis of COPD and cor pulmonale, has started on a diuretic and 3L of oxygen. In the physician's clinical notes, pulmonary hypertension and polycythemia are noted.

21. The diuretic therapy is done to provide all of the following benefits *except*:
    A. reduce lower extremity edema.
    B. improve right ventricular function.
    C. improve ambulation.
    D. increase circulating volume.

22. In preparing for the setup of oxygen therapy for Mr. Crowne, you would bring a flow meter and:
    A. nasal cannula.
    B. nasal cannula and humidifier.
    C. simple mask.
    D. simple mask and humidifier.

23. Several days later, Mr. Crowne's condition has improved. His doctor asks you to evaluate Mr. Crowne for long-term oxygen therapy at home. All of the following would be indicative of long-term oxygen therapy *except*:
    A. right-sided heart failure.
    B. pulmonary hypertension.
    C. hematocrit of 60%.
    D. PaO_2 of 60 mm Hg at rest and on room air.

24. _____ vaccination has been beneficial in the reduction of morbidity in patients with COPD; therefore, it is recommended for these patients.
    A. Viral
    B. Pneumococcal
    C. Streptococcal
    D. Staphylococcal

25. The best way to hydrate and thin airway secretions is to provide:
    A. oral fluid intake.
    B. surface active agents.
    C. intravenous fluid.
    D. aerosol therapy.

26. Overlap syndrome describes the coexistence of COPD and _____. The mainstay therapy for this condition is _____.
    A. obstructive sleep apnea; CPAP
    B. obstructive sleep apnea; mechanical ventilation
    C. central sleep apnea; CPAP
    D. central sleep apnea; mechanical ventilation

27. Exercise training, patient and family education, instruction in respiratory care procedures, and psychologic support are components of a typical _____ program.
    A. cardiac rehabilitation
    B. pulmonary rehabilitation
    C. exercise training
    D. exercise conditioning

28. Bullectomy:
    A. is done to compress healthy lung tissue.
    B. is done to compress large bullae.
    C. involves removal of healthy lung tissue.
    D. involves removal of large bullae.

29. Lung volume reduction surgery:
    A. generally removes 40 to 50% of lung tissue.
    B. decreases elastic recoil of remaining lung.
    C. enhances pulmonary mechanics.
    D. improves left ventricular function.

30. Lung volume reduction surgery is helpful in restoring the lung function of patients with:
    A. emphysema.
    B. a long smoking history.
    C. hyperactive airways.
    D. restrictive lung disease.

31. The inclusive criteria for lung transplantation include:
    A. patients over 65 years of age.
    B. an FEV_1 less than 25%.
    C. presence of congestive heart failure.
    D. continuing use of cigarettes.

32. The management strategies to alleviate acute exacerbation of the patients with COPD include all of the following *except*:
    A. intubation and mechanical ventilation in life-threatening respiratory failure.
    B. use of steroids for severe exacerbation.
    C. oxygen therapy to maintain adequate oxygenation.
    D. avoidance of $ß_2$-agonists and anticholinergic medications.

33. Based on the American Thoracic Society (ATS) recommended guidelines:
    A. peak flow values are predictor of need for hospitalization.
    B. peak flow values may be used to determine readiness for discharge.
    C. $ß_2$-agonists should be given with a metered-dose inhaler.
    D. inhaled anticholinergics should not be mixed with $ß_2$-agonists.

34. Solu-Medrol is a _____ and it may help to improve the _____ values in hospitalized patients with acute exacerbation of COPD.
    A. methylxanthine; spirometry
    B. methylxanthine; blood gas
    C. steroid; blood gas
    D. steroid; spirometry

35. Dr. King asks you to start oxygen therapy for Mr. Lambert, a patient with COPD and mild exacerbation. You would start and titrate the oxygen flow until _____ is obtained.
    A. SpO_2 of 60%
    B. SpO_2 of 95%
    C. pO_2 of 60 mm Hg
    D. pO_2 of 95 mm Hg

36. When patients with COPD are treated with noninvasive positive pressure ventilation (NPPV), a _____ is found.
    A. higher mortality rate
    B. higher incidence of intubation
    C. lower incidence of mechanical ventilation
    D. all of the above

Questions 37 to 40: Match the modes or settings used during mechanical ventilation in Column I with the rationales in Column II. Use each answer ONCE.

Column I	Column II
37. Assist-control	A. To reduce work of breathing due to tubing airflow resistance
38. SIMV	B. To alleviate respiratory work in extremely fatigued patients
39. Pressure support	C. To prevent air trapping
40. Short inspiratory time	D. To avoid respiratory muscle atrophy

Questions 41 to 46: Mr. Davidson, a patient with COPD, is suffering from acute ventilatory failure and is being mechanically ventilated. His physician writes an order "respiratory care to manage ventilator."

41. While you are assessing Mr. Davidson and his ventilator, you notice that the ventilator registers an auto-PEEP of 6 cm H_2O. This condition is related to _____ and the problem may be solved by _____.
    A. insufficient expiratory time; increasing the inspiratory time
    B. insufficient expiratory time; using a larger tidal volume
    C. air trapping; using a higher respiratory rate
    D. air trapping; using a lower tidal volume

42. After trying the strategy that you have selected in the preceding question, the auto-PEEP remains at 6 cm H_2O. You would use an applied _____ of _____ cm H_2O.
    A. PEEP; 5
    B. PEEP; 6
    C. pressure support; 5
    D. pressure support; 6

43. Three days later, Mr. Davidson's condition has improved and you are trying to determine his readiness to wean from mechanical ventilation. The most sensitive predictor of weaning success is the:
    A. arterial blood gases (ABGs).
    B. rapid shallow breathing index (RSBI).
    C. maximal inspiratory pressure (MIP).
    D. forced vital capacity (FVC).

44. To measure the parameter you have selected in the preceding question, you would need to obtain Mr. Davidson's:
    A. arterial blood sample.
    B. spontaneous tidal volume and respiratory rate.
    C. negative pressure reading during inspiratory occlusion.
    D. pulmonary function results.

45. Mr. Davidson is ready for the weaning trial when his:
    A. $PaCO_2$ is greater than 60 mm Hg.
    B. PaO_2 is less than 50 mm Hg.
    C. RSBI is greater than 110.
    D. RSBI is less than 100.

46. To begin weaning Mr. Davidson, you would use _____ weaning.
    A. inverse ratio
    B. pressure control
    C. CPAP (continuous positive airway pressure)
    D. pressure support

47. Advance directives such as living will or durable powers of attorney for heath care are terms associated with:
    A. mechanical ventilation.
    B. patients with COPD.
    C. end-of-life care.
    D. patient education.

48. Patients with COPD may qualify for hospice services when they meet all of the following conditions *except*:
    A. presence of cor pulmonale.
    B. disabling dyspnea at rest.
    C. pCO_2 50 mm Hg or higher.
    D. SpO_2 95% or lower.

Questions 49 to 52: Refer to the case studies in this chapter and match the patient findings in Column I with the supporting laboratory results or patient characteristics in Column II. Use each answer ONCE.

Column I	Column II
49. Air flow obstruction	A. Increased $PaCO_2$
	B. Use of accessory muscles during spontaneous breathing
50. Hyperinflation of lung	
51. Hypoventilation	C. FEV_1 of 65% predicted normal
52. Shortness of breath and increased work of breathing	D. Increased RV, FRC, and TLC

CHAPTER 48

Interstitial Lung Disease

1. Interstitial lung disease (ILD) is characterized by the _____ in the interstitium of the lung parenchyma.
   A. inflammation or fibrosis or both
   B. edema or atelectasis or both
   C. consolidation or edema or both
   D. edema or inflammation or both

2. The key diagnostic features of ILD include:
   I. dyspnea at rest or on exertion.
   II. bilateral diffuse infiltrates on chest radiograph.
   III. obstructive lung defects.
   IV. restrictive lung defects.
   A. I, II, and IV
   B. I, III, and IV
   C. II and III
   D. II and IV

3. The definitive diagnosis of ILD is made with a:
   A. chest radiograph.
   B. pulmonary function study.
   C. detailed history and physical.
   D. biopsy.

4. Mr. Carlton has an admitting diagnosis of shortness of breath with unknown etiology. Tests are being done to rule out ILD. Which of the following pulmonary function results would correlate with a diagnosis of ILD?
   A. Increase in lung volumes and capacities
   B. Decrease in flow rates
   C. Decrease in diffusion capacity
   D. All of the above

5. Interstitial lung diseases share a similar pathophysiology. Arrange the following structural changes in a correct order of development.
   I. Fibrous tissue
   II. Alveolitis and vasculitis
   III. Collagen and connective tissue elements
   IV. Alveolar, capillary, and parenchymal cell injury
   A. I, III, IV, II
   B. II, IV, III, I
   C. III, II, I, IV
   D. IV, II, I, III

Questions 6 to 10: Match the classifications of ILD in Column I with the respective examples in Column II. Use each answer ONCE.

Column I	Column II
6. Infection	A. Silicosis, pneumo-coniosis
7. Occupational exposure	B. Narcotics, nonsteroidal antiinflammatory drugs
8. Neoplasm	C. Bacterial, viral, fungal pneumonia
9. Congenital and metabolic causes	D. Cystic fibrosis, lipoid-oses
10. Drug reactions	E. Bronchoalveolar carci-noma, leukemia

11. The most common clinical manifestation of ILD is a gradual onset of _____ along with a _____ cough.
    A. pneumonia; productive
    B. pneumonia; nonproductive
    C. dyspnea; productive
    D. dyspnea; nonproductive

12. For patients with interstitial lung disease, all of the following pulmonary function results would be lower than normal *except*:
    A. total lung capacity.
    B. FEV_1 and FVC.
    C. FEV_1/FVC ratio.
    D. diffusion capacity.

13. For patients with interstitial lung disease, the FEV_1/FVC ratio is _____ because _____.
    A. increased; FEV_1 is increased and FVC is decreased
    B. near normal; both FEV_1 and FVC are increased
    C. near normal; both FEV_1 and FVC are decreased
    D. decreased; FEV_1 is decreased and FVC is increased

14. The diagnosis of ILD often requires different methods of evaluation. Arrange the following methods of evaluation in a correct order, from simple to complex.
    I. Bronchoscopy
    II. History, physical exam, PFTs, lab studies
    III. High-resolution CT scan
    IV. Open lung biopsy
    V. Chest radiographs
    A. I, II, III, V, IV
    B. II, V, III, I, IV
    C. III, II, I, V, IV
    D. V, III, I, II, IV

15. _____ is considered the gold standard for a specific diagnosis of ILD.
    A. Lung biopsy
    B. Bronchoalveolar lavage
    C. High-resolution computed tomography
    D. Pulmonary function study

16. Factors indicating an improved prognosis in idiopathic pulmonary fibrosis include all of the following *except*:
    A. greater cellular response in lavage.
    B. less dyspneic condition.
    C. younger age.
    D. male patient.

Questions 17 to 20. Match the conditions associated with ILD in Column I with the respective supportive measures in Column II. Use each answer ONCE.

Column I	Column II
17. Alveolitis	A. Bronchodilators
	B. Oxygen therapy
18. Frequent purulent sputum	C. Antibiotics
	D. Corticosteroid or
19. Wheezing	immunosuppressive
	agents
20. Hypoxemia	

21. _____ is the most common disease associated with ILD characterized by development of nonceseating granulomas in two or more organ systems.
    A. Idiopathic pulmonary fibrosis
    B. Sarcoidosis
    C. Collagen vascular disease
    D. Pulmonary alveolar proteinosis

CHAPTER 49

Pulmonary Vascular Disease

1. Pulmonary circulation is a _____, high-flow system that provides very _____ flow resistance to the blood coming from the right ventricle.
   A. low-pressure; high
   B. low-pressure; low
   C. high-pressure; high
   D. high-pressure; low

2. An increase in pulmonary vascular resistance or pulmonary hypertension may develop in all of the following conditions *except*:
   A. destruction or obliteration of the pulmonary blood vessels.
   B. obstruction of the pulmonary blood flow.
   C. hypoxic vasoconstriction.
   D. hypovolemia.

3. Mr. Hanks, a patient with long-standing pulmonary hypertension, is admitted for severe shortness of breath. If his condition is worsen or left untreated, the most likely pathophysiological finding may be:
   A. a decreased pulmonary artery pressure.
   B. a reduced right ventricle afterload.
   C. left ventricular failure.
   D. enlargement of the right ventricle.

Questions 4 to 8: Match the causes of pulmonary hypertension in Column I with the respective diagnoses in Column II. Use each answer ONCE.

Column I

4. Obstruction of the pulmonary vasculature

5. Pulmonary parenchymal disease

6. Cardiac disease

7. Intrinsic disorders of the pulmonary vasculature

8. Pulmonary hypertension associated with systemic

Column II

A. COPD, interstitial lung disease
B. Drugs, crack cocaine
C. HIV, sleep apnea
D. Venous thromboembolism, sickle cell disease
E. Left-sided heart failure, left-sided valvular disease

9. In acute pulmonary embolism, hypoxemia occurs due to _____ ventilation/perfusion ratio or _____.
   A. high; dead space ventilation
   B. high; intrapulmonary shunting
   C. low; dead space ventilation
   D. low; intrapulmonary shunting

10. When the pulmonary artery pressure approaches _____ mm Hg, the right ventricle may not be able to generate an adequate systolic pressure to sustain the workload. The end result will be heart failure and death.
    A. 20
    B. 30
    C. 40
    D. 50

Questions 11 to 13: A patient is brought to the emergency room with severe tachypnea and tachycardia. Preliminary physical exam suggests pulmonary embolism.

11. Which of the following is not a risk factor for this diagnosis?
    A. Recent surgery
    B. Immobilization/paralysis
    C. Pneumonia
    D. Malignancy

12. Which of the following noninvasive tests should be done to rule out pulmonary embolism?
    A. Ventilation/perfusion scan
    B. Pulmonary angiogram
    C. Chest radiography
    D. Arterial blood gases

13. If the test in the preceding question is inconclusive for this diagnosis, _____ should be considered.
    A. flexible bronchoscopy
    B. open lung biopsy
    C. pulmonary angiogram
    D. ventilation/perfusion scan

14. A loud _____ valve closure sound is common characteristic in patients with pulmonary hypertension.
    A. mitral
    B. pulmonic
    C. tricuspid
    D. aortic

15. The gold standard for the diagnosis of pulmonary hypertension is:
    A. pulmonary angiogram.
    B. ventilation/perfusion scan.
    C. right heart catheterization.
    D. left heart catheterization.

16. Once a diagnosis of pulmonary embolism is made, a(n) _____ such as _____ should be started immediately.
    A. anticoagulant; heparin
    B. bronchodilator; albuterol
    C. chronotropic agent; epinephrine
    D. vasodilator; morphine sulfate

17. _____ is one of the serious complications of prolonged heparin therapy.
    A. Kidney failure
    B. Liver failure
    C. Bleeding
    D. Heart failure

18. In the management of cor pulmonale, oxygen therapy should be started when the patient's PaO_2 is _____ mm Hg or less.
    A. 50
    B. 60
    C. 70
    D. 80

19. Calcium channel blockers, Prostacyclin, and anticoagulants have been used successfully in the management of:
    A. primary pulmonary hypertension.
    B. secondary pulmonary hypertension.
    C. pulmonary embolism.
    D. cor pulmonale.

20. Prostacyclin is a pulmonary _____ and it is effective in the treatment of patients with _____.
    A. bronchodilator; pulmonary embolism
    B. bronchodilator; pulmonary hypertension
    C. vasodilator; pulmonary embolism
    B. vasodilator; pulmonary hypertension

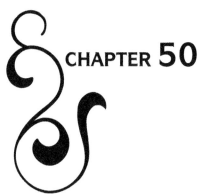

CHAPTER 50

Pneumonia

1. Pneumonia is the inflammation and consolidation of the lung tissue caused by:
   A. microbes.
   B. dust and pollens.
   C. chemicals.
   D. infectious agents.

2. Mr. Crawford has been mechanically ventilated for one week and his most recent chest radiograph shows bilateral consolidation in the lower lobes. You have also suctioned a moderate amount of purulent secretions from his endotracheal tube. Mr. Crawford's condition may be described as:
   A. early-onset hospital-acquired pneumonia.
   B. late-onset hospital-acquired pneumonia.
   C. early-onset ventilator-associated pneumonia.
   B. late-onset ventilator-associated pneumonia.

Questions 3 to 5: Match the types of pneumonia in Column I with the probable causes in Column II. Use each answer ONCE.

Column I

Column II

3. Primary endogenous pneumonias

4. Secondary endogenous pneumonias

5. Exogenous pneumonias

A. Hospital-acquired, commonly caused by organisms colonizing respiratory care equipment and supplies

B. Usually hospital-acquired, commonly caused by *Pseudomonas aeruginosa* and *Enterobacter* species

C. Usually community-acquired, commonly caused by *Streptococcus pneumoniae* and *Hemophilus influenzae*

6. Gram staining or culturing of sputum samples may not accurately reveal the organisms causing the pneumonia due to:
   A. contamination of sample during collection.
   B. treatment with antibiotics before collection.
   C. inadequate collection method.
   D. all of the above.

7. _____ is needed to exclude empyema or complicated parapneumonic effusion in patients with a primary diagnosis of pneumonia.
   A. Blood culture
   B. Pleural fluid
   C. Serology
   D. Sputum culture and sensitivity

8. Samples obtained by bronchoalveolar lavage (BAL) may be used for all of the following studies *except:*
   A. serology.
   B. bacterial culture.
   C. *Pneumocystis*, mycobacterial, and fungal stains.
   D. cytology.

9. *Streptococcus pneumoniae*, *Staphylococcus aureus*, and *Enterococcus* species are:
   A. gram-positive fungi.
   B. gram-positive bacteria.
   C. gram-negative fungi.
   D. gram-negative bacteria.

10. Third-generation cephalosporins, imipenem, and vancomycin are _____ used to treat pneumonia caused by _____.
    A. corticosteroids; *Streptococcus pneumoniae*
    B. corticosteroids; penicillin-resistant *Streptococcus pneumoniae*
    C. antibiotics; *Streptococcus pneumoniae*
    B. antibiotics; penicillin-resistant *Streptococcus pneumoniae*

11. Pneumonia caused by *Streptococcus pneumoniae* usually produces _____-colored sputum, whereas the sputum in *Staphylococcus aureus* infections is _____ in character.
    A. rusty; foamy
    B. rusty; purulent (pus)
    C. white; foamy
    D. white; purulent (pus)

12. *Haemophilus influenzae, Moraxella catarrhalis, Pseudomonas aeruginosa, Klebsiella* species, *Escherichia coli*, and *Enterobacter* species are examples of:
    A. gram-positive bacteria.
    B. gram-positive fungi.
    C. gram-negative bacteria.
    D. gram-negative fungi.

13. _____ is isolated most often in ventilator-associated pneumonia and it is the leading cause of death among intubated patients with pneumonia.
    A. *Haemophilus influenzae*
    B. *Klebsiella* species
    C. *Escherichia coli*
    D. *Pseudomonas aeruginosa*

Questions 14 to 18: Match the atypical organisms responsible for pneumonia in Column I with the associated reservoirs in Column II. You may use any answer MORE THAN ONCE.

Column I

14. *Legionellosis*

15. *Mycoplasma pneumoniae*

16. *Chlamydia psittaci*

17. *Chlamydia pneumoniae*

18. *Coxiella burnetii*

Column II

A. Military camps, boarding schools
B. Domestic water and wet cooling systems
C. Cattle
D. Birds and bird products

19. Anaerobic bacterial infection is usually caused by _____.
    A. aspiration of stomach contents
    B. aspiration of oropharyngeal secretions
    C. fungal infection
    D. gram-negative infection

20. Aerosolized ribavirin is used to treat the _____ infection caused by _____.
    A. fungal; *Varicella zoster*
    B. fungal; herpes simplex
    C. viral; respiratory syncytial virus
    D. viral; parainfluenza

21. *Acid fast smear, purified protein derivative (PPD) skin test, isoniazid,* and *rifampin* are terms related to pneumonia caused by _____ infection.
    A. mycobacterial
    B. fungal
    C. viral
    D. atypical bacterial

Questions 22 to 27: Match the types of fungal respiratory infection in Column I with the characteristics in Column II. Use each answer ONCE.

Column I

22. Histoplasmosis

23. Blastomycosis

24. Coccidioidomycosis

25. Cryptococcosis

26. Aspergillosis

27. Candidiasis

Column II

A. Common where molds are found (soil, dust, and water), acquired by inhalation
B. Common in southwestern United States and some countries of South America, found in soil in arid and semiarid climates, acquired by inhalation
C. Common in Ohio and Mississippi River valleys, found in avian (bird) droppings
D. Found in soil, food, gastrointestinal tract, skin, and hospital environment, may be acquired in hospital
E. Common in southern and upper midwestern United States, found in decaying organic matters, acquired sexually or by inhalation
F. Worldwide distribution, found in avian droppings, acquired by inhalation

28. With community-acquired pneumonia:
    A. patients should be treated in the hospital.
    B. antibiotics are started after confirmation by sputum culture.
    C. common pathogens include S. *Pneumoniae,* H. *Influenzae,* and influenza A virus.
    D. severity is not associated with coexisting conditions.

29. With hospital-acquired pneumonia:
    A. the mortality rate is less than 10%.
    B. patients with different severity respond to the same antibiotics.
    C. surveillance and infection control programs are essential in reducing its incidence.
    D. *Pseudomonas aeruginosa* and MRSA are two common early-onset pathogens.

30. In immunocompromised patients with pneumonia:
    A. sputum culture is often diagnostic of pathogens involved.
    B. coexisting pulmonary infections are rare.
    C. pathogens causing pneumonia may include bacteria, mycobacteria, fungi, and viruses.
    D. all of the above.

31. *Pneumocystis carinii* pneumonia is often seen in patients:
    A. with HIV.
    B. with tuberculosis.
    C. who are young and healthy.
    D. who are being mechanically ventilated.

32. Pneumonia in children is more problematic because they have smaller airways, _____ compliant thoracic cages, and underdeveloped _____.
    A. more; immune systems
    B. more; lungs
    C. less; immune systems
    D. less; lungs

CHAPTER 51

Cystic Fibrosis

1. Cystic fibrosis is the most lethal _____ disease in the _____ population.
   A. genetic; Caucasian
   B. genetic; non-Caucasian
   C. infectious; Caucasian
   D. infectious; non-Caucasian

2. Cystic fibrosis transmembrane conductance regulator (CFTR) is the _____ responsible for cystic fibrosis.
   A. chromosome
   B. blood type
   C. gene
   D. carrier

3. Cystic fibrosis is inherited in an autosomal _____ pattern and carriers of the mutated CFTR gene _____ have any symptoms of cystic fibrosis.
   A. dominant; do
   B. dominant; do not
   C. recessive; do
   D. recessive; do not

4. When one of the parents is a carrier of cystic fibrosis, the child will have a _____ chance of becoming a carrier.
   A. 25%
   B. 50%
   C. 75%
   D. 100%

5. When one of the parents is a carrier of cystic fibrosis, the child will have a _____ chance of becoming affected by cystic fibrosis.
   A. 0%
   B. 25%
   C. 50%
   D. 100%

6. In cystic fibrosis with the mutated CFTR genes, the epithelial ion transfer is _____ because normal CFTR regulates several ion conductance pathways. This condition _____ the host defense.
   A. enhanced; strengthens
   B. enhanced; weakens
   C. hindered; strengthens
   D. hindered; weakens

7. In the lung, the absence of normal CFTR results in _____ hyperabsorption from the airway lumen and a diminished capacity to secrete _____ via CFTR. This leads to reduced airway clearance and eventual airway obstruction and bacterial infection.
   A. sodium; bicarbonate
   B. sodium; chloride
   C. chloride; potassium
   D. chloride; magnesium

8. Methods for the diagnosis of cystic fibrosis include all of the following *except*:
   A. clinical features consistent with cystic fibrosis.
   B. sweat testing.
   C. sputum analysis.
   D. CFTR mutational analyses.

Questions 9 to 14: Match the organ or system involvement in cystic fibrosis in Column I with the clinical manifestations in Column II. Use each answer ONCE.

Column I

9. Upper respiratory tract

10. Exocrine and endocrine pancreas

11. Gastrointestinal tract

12. Hepatobiliary system

13. Reproductive tract

14. Sweat glands

Column II

A. Impaired absorption of fat-soluble vitamins, recurrent pancreatitis, diabetes

B. High chloride concentration in sweat

C. Infertility in males due to obstruction of the vas deferens

D. Recurrence of nasal polyps and sinus symptoms

E. Colon obstruction, constipation

F. Persistent elevation of liver enzymes

Questions 15 to 19: Mr. Howard, a 29-year-old patient with cystic fibrosis, has been admitted to the medical floor for pneumonia and acute exacerbation. You are assigned to provide respiratory care.

15. In reviewing Mr. Howard's chest radiograph, you are likely to see:
    A. hyperinflation.
    B. cystic bronchiectasis.
    C. increased interstitial markings.
    D. all of the above.

16. Mr. Howard's pulmonary function study may reveal an increased:
    A. FEV_1.
    B. RV/TLC.
    C. $FEV_{25-75\%}$.
    D. FVC.

17. In Mr. Howard's laboratory report, the pathogen cultured from the sputum is most likely:
    A. *Pseudomonas aeruginosa*.
    B. *Staphylococcus aureus*.
    C. *Burkholderia cepacia*.
    D. *Mycobacterium avium*.

18. Of the pathogens identified in the preceding question, _____ may spread from person to person and cause a rapid clinical decline with fever and sepsis.
    A. *Pseudomonas aeruginosa*.
    B. *Staphylococcus aureus*.
    C. *Burkholderia cepacia*.
    D. *Mycobacterium avium*.

19. About 12 hours following admission, Mr. Howard becomes extremely agitated and chest radiograph at this time shows a 30% pneumothorax. The treatment for this condition should be:
    A. clinical monitoring and oxygen therapy.
    B. bronchial artery embolization.
    C. tube thoracostomy.
    D. mechanical ventilation.

20. For cystic fibrosis patients with hypoxemia and hypercapnia, the *initial* treatment strategy should involve all of the following *except*:
    A. oxygen therapy.
    B. mechanical ventilation.
    C. antibiotics.
    D. secretion mobilization.

Questions 21 to 25: Match the types of airway maintenance therapy for cystic fibrosis in Column I with the clinical examples in Column II. Use each answer ONCE.

Column I

21. Remove secretions

22. Modifier characteristic of secretions

23. Treat infection

24. Reduce airflow resistance

25. Reduce inflammation

Column II

A. Tobramycin, colistin

B. Beta-adrenergics and anticholinergics

C. Corticosteroids, high-dose ibuprofen

D. Pulmozyme, Mucomyst, hypertonic saline

E. Chest physiotherapy, positive expiratory pressure (PEP) device, flutter valve

26. Lung transplantation is suitable for _____ CF lung disease in which the _____ is less than 30% predicted normal.
    A. early-stage; $FEF_{25-75\%}$.
    B. early-stage; FEV_1.
    C. end-stage; $FEF_{25-75\%}$.
    D. end-stage; FEV_1.

CHAPTER 52

Acute Respiratory Distress Syndrome

1. In acute respiratory distress syndrome (ARDS), severe hypoxemia is quantified by a _____ ratio of _____ mm Hg or less.
   A. PaO_2/F_IO_2; 200
   B. PaO_2/F_IO_2; 300
   C. PaO_2/P_AO_2; 200
   D. PaO_2/P_AO_2; 300

2. A PaO_2/F_IO_2 ratio of 200 mm Hg or less is one of the characteristics used by the American-European Consensus Conference (AECC) to define presence of:
   A. chronic obstructive pulmonary disease.
   B. acute lung injury.
   C. chronic ventilatory failure.
   D. ARDS.

3. The most reliable indicator of the severity of ARDS is the:
   B. chest radiography finding.
   A. PaO_2/F_IO_2 ratio.
   C. pulmonary artery wedge pressure measurement.
   D. lung compliance measurement.

Questions 4 to 7. Match the clinical conditions in Column I with the type of risk factor for ARDS in Column II. You may use any answer MORE THAN ONCE.

Column I

4. Pneumonia

5. Sepsis

6. Aspiration of gastric contents

7. Lung contusion

Column II

A. Direct lung injury

B. Indirect lung injury

Questions 8 to 9. You are called to the medical intensive care unit to perform an elective intubation on Ms. Busbee, a patient with a diagnosis of ARDS.

8. In assessing Ms. Busbee's condition, you would likely see all of the following findings *except:*
   A. rapid shallow breathing pattern.
   B. increased lung compliance.
   C. bilateral opacities on chest radiograph.
   D. reduced PaO_2/F_IO_2 ratio.

9. Ms. Busbee's severe hypoxemia may be attributed to all of the following pathophysiologic changes *except:*
   A. ventilation/perfusion mismatch.
   B. intrapulmonary shunting.
   C. hyperventilation.
   D. pulmonary capillary permeability.

10. The result of the fibroproliferative phase of ARDS may be right heart failure. Arrange the following events in correct sequence leading to right heart failure, starting from the earliest.
    I. Pulmonary hypertension
    II. Fibrosis formation
    III. Destruction of pulmonary capillaries
    A. I, II, III
    B. I, III, II
    C. II, III, I
    D. III, II, I

11. In the early stage of ARDS, destruction of the type 1 alveolar epithelial cells leads to a(n):
    A. increased permeability and pulmonary edema.
    B. decreased permeability and atelectasis.
    C. increased alveolar ventilation and respiratory alkalosis.
    D. decreased pulmonary artery pressure and hypoperfusion.

12. Development of hydrostatic pulmonary edema in ARDS is related to:
    A. oxygen toxicity.
    B. mechanical ventilation.
    C. overdistention of the lungs.
    D. heart failure.

13. Management of ARDS includes avoidance of ICU-related complications such as:
    A. ventilator-associated pneumonia.
    B. deep vein thrombosis.
    C. gastritis.
    D. all of the above.

14. Surfactant replacement in ARDS _____ therapeutic because any remaining surfactant in adult lungs is _____.
    A. is; functional
    B. is; capable of increasing surface tension
    C. is not; dysfunctional.
    D. is not; likely to decrease surface function

15. Prone positioning has been used successfully to improve the _____ status of patients with ARDS.
    A. oxygenation
    B. ventilation
    C. hemodynamic
    D. A and B

16. The effective ventilator strategies include _____ to maintain alveolar recruitment and _____ tidal volume to protect lungs.
    A. PEEP; high
    B. PEEP; low
    C. high pressure; high
    D. high; low

17. Positive end-expiratory pressure (PEEP) helps to:
    A. decrease functional residual capacity.
    B. increase intrapulmonary shunting.
    C. decrease compliance.
    D. recruit alveoli.

18. Prior to weaning the PEEP, the patient's hemodynamic status must be stable and the PaO_2 should be at least _____ mm Hg on F_IO_2 of _____% or less.
    A. 60; 40
    B. 60; 60
    C. 80; 40
    D. 80; 60

19. Weaning of PEEP may continue if the PaO_2 at a lower PEEP decreases by less than _____% from the prewean PaO_2.
    A. 20
    B. 30
    C. 40
    D. 50

20. In using the lung-protective strategy on patients with acute lung injury, the tidal volume is initially set at _____ mL/kg with a plateau pressure target of less than _____ cm H_2O.
    A. 6; 20
    B. 6; 30
    C. 10; 20
    D. 10; 30

21. In the chapter case study "ARDS After Multiple Trauma," the patient's pulmonary edema _____ likely due to heart failure because the _____.
    A. is; P/F ratio is 100 mm Hg
    B. is not; P/F ratio is 100 mm Hg
    C. is; PAWP is 16 mm Hg
    D. is not; PAWP is 16 mm Hg

CHAPTER 53

Postoperative Respiratory Care

1. Preoperative patient assessment is done to:
   A. minimize complications during and after surgery.
   B. guide the use of proper anesthesia.
   C. alleviate risk factors.
   D. all of the above.

2. Mr. Jamison, a 65-year-old patient, has been scheduled to have coronary artery bypass graft (CABG) surgery. In reviewing his medical record, you notice the following patient conditions. Which of these are considered risk factors for postoperative pulmonary complications?

   I. Age
   II. History of cardiac disease
   III. 160 lbs, 5'11"
   IV. Room air PaO_2 = 55 mm Hg

   A. I and II
   B. I and IV
   C. II, III, and IV
   D. II and IV

3. The elective surgery scheduled for Ms. Lange has been postponed due to increased risk of postoperative complications. In order to reduce her risk, Ms. Lange should do all of the following *except*:
   A. start a high-protein diet.
   B. stop smoking for at least eight weeks.
   C. reduce excessive body weight.
   D. use bronchodilators and steroids as prescribed.

4. Total parenteral nutrition (TPN) is a method of feeding intended for:
   A. patients with cardiac disease.
   B. patients with pulmonary disease.
   C. malnourished patients.
   D. obese patients.

5. Preoperative testing should include _____ for patients with COPD.
   A. arterial blood gases
   B. electrocardiogram
   C. chest radiograph
   D. All of the above

Questions 6 to 10. Match the clinical conditions in Column I with the suggested preoperative tests in Column II. You may use any answer MORE THAN ONCE.

Column I

6. Tracheal deviation

7. Hypertension

8. Hypoxemia

9. Pneumonia

10. Chest pain

Column II

A. Arterial blood gases
B. Electrocardiogram
C. Chest radiograph

11. Which of the following procedures carries the highest intraoperative risk and risk for postoperative pulmonary complications?
    A. Endotracheal intubation
    B. Thoracic surgery
    C. Lower abdominal surgery
    D. Insertion of pulmonary artery catheter

12. Intraoperative blood loss of _____ mL or more is likely to increase the incidence of pulmonary complications.
    A. 300
    B. 600
    C. 1200
    D. 2400

13. Mechanical ventilation is used to support patients with _____ following surgery.
    A. persistent hypercapnia
    B. nutritional deficit
    C. severe pain
    D. diminished muscle strength

14. Five-second head-lift or leg-lift is done to assess a patient's _____ following surgery.
    A. mental status
    B. muscle strength
    C. task orientation
    D. nutritional status

15. Which of the following is not a sign or finding of atelectasis?
    A. Air trapping
    B. Inspiratory crackles or diminished breath sounds
    C. Mediastinal shift
    D. Tachycardia and hypoxemia

16. Atelectasis leads to:
    A. dead space ventilation.
    B. hyperventilation.
    C. left to right shunt.
    D. right to left shunt.

17. Pulmonary embolism may exhibit all of the following signs or findings *except:*
    A. wheezing or crackles.
    B. respiratory acidosis.
    C. tachypnea and dyspnea.
    D. ventilation/perfusion mismatch.

18. Ventilation/perfusion scan and pulmonary angiography are used to diagnose:
    A. pulmonary embolism.
    B. atelectasis.
    C. pneumonia.
    D. all of the above.

19. Which of the following is not a sign or condition of pneumonia?
    A. Purulent sputum production
    B. Leukocytosis
    C. Mediastinal shift
    D. Fever

20. Selection of proper antibiotics should be guided by the results of _____ of sputum sample.
    A. acid fast stain
    B. gram stain
    C. microscopic examination
    D. culture and sensitivity

21. For postoperative respiratory care, mechanical ventilation is used as a supporting measure for the:
    A. residual effect of anesthesia.
    B. induced respiratory depression following neurosurgery.
    C. surgical trauma following thoracic procedures.
    D. all of the above.

CHAPTER **54**

Cardiac Failure

1. Cardiac failure occurs when the heart cannot meet the metabolic needs of the _____ and this condition is most common in _____ patients.
   A. tissues; trauma
   B. tissues; elderly
   C. heart; trauma
   D. heart; elderly

2. Some common etiologies of cardiac failure include all of the following *except*:
   A. alcohol.
   B. idiopathic dilated cardiomyopathy.
   C. hypotension.
   D. coronary artery disease.

3. _____ is the smallest unit of heart muscle that contracts.
   A. Myocyte
   B. Sarcomere
   C. Myofibril
   D. Troponin

4. Multiple _____ make up a myofibril and each muscle cell (myocyte) contains numerous myofibrils.
   A. troponin
   B. H bands
   C. mitochondria
   D. sarcomeres

5. Contraction of the myocyte is initiated by cell membrane:
   A. depolarization.
   B. repolarization.
   C. dissociation.
   D. association.

6. The sarcoplasmic reticulum initiates contraction by releasing _____ ions into the cytoplasm.
   A. hydrogen
   B. calcium
   C. potassium
   D. sodium

7. In the presence of calcium, the sarcomeres _____ and lead to _____ of the myocytes.
   A. lengthen; contraction
   B. lengthen; relaxation
   C. shorten; contraction
   D. shorten; relaxation

8. The normal stroke volume is about _____ mL and it is usually _____ than the left ventricular end-diastolic volume (LVEDV).
   A. 60 to 70; larger
   B. 60 to 70; smaller
   C. 80 to 100; larger
   D. 80 to 100; smaller

9. Stroke volume is reduced when the venous return is _____ or the downstream vascular resistance is _____.
   A. increased; increased
   B. increased; decreased
   C. decreased; increased
   D. decreased; decreased

10. The opening or closure of the aortic valve is mainly dependent on the pressure gradient between the:
    A. pulmonary artery and left ventricle.
    B. pulmonary artery and right ventricle.
    C. aorta and left ventricle.
    D. aorta and right ventricle.

11. Diastolic filling of the ventricles occurs:
    I. following systole.
    II. during relaxation of the ventricles.
    III. during contraction of the atria.
    A. I
    B. I and II
    C. II
    D. I, II, and III

12. Ventricular function is determined by the:
    A. contractility.
    B. preload.
    C. afterload.
    D. all of the above.

13. The ß-adrenergic receptors, adenylate cyclase and _____, affect the contractility of the heart because they alter the release and reuptake of _____ in the cytoplasm. [cAMP: cyclic adenosine monophosphate; cGMP: cyclic guanine monophosphate]
    A. cAMP; calcium
    B. cGMP; sodium
    C. cAMP and cGMP; calcium
    D. cAMP and cGMP; sodium

Questions 14 to 18: Match the pathophysiology of heart failure in Column I with the clinical examples in Column II. Use each answer ONCE.

Column I

14. Restricted filling

15. Pressure overload

16. Volume overload

17. Contractile impairment

18. Arrhythmia

Column II

A. Mitral/tricuspid stenosis, tamponade

B. Ischemia, dilated cardiomyopathy

C. Pulmonary hypertension, aortic/pulmonary stenosis

D. Tachycardia, bradycardia

E. Valvular regurgitation, ventricular septal defect

19. In progressive aortic regurgitation, the:
    A. true forward stroke volume is increased.
    B. LVEDV is reduced.
    C. wall of LV becomes thinner gradually.
    D. heart enlarges gradually.

20. Failure of the cardiac muscle to relax normally (diastolic dysfunction) results in _____ filling pressures and symptoms of _____ congestion despite normal systolic function.
    A. increased; pulmonary
    B. increased; pulmonary and systemic
    C. decreased; pulmonary
    D. decreased; pulmonary and systemic

21. Forward heart failure is a condition in which the _____ do not receive _____ blood flow from the heart.
    A. pulmonary blood vessels; pulmonary
    B. pulmonary blood vessels; adequate
    C. organs; systemic
    D. organs; adequate

22. In general, left ventricular failure causes _____ congestion of the _____ circulation.
    A. arterial; systemic
    B. arterial; pulmonary
    C. venous; systemic
    D. venous; pulmonary

23. Mr. Hamm has an admitting diagnosis of cor pulmonale (right-sided heart failure). This condition often leads to _____ congestion of the _____ circulation.
    A. arterial; systemic
    B. arterial; pulmonary
    C. venous; systemic
    D. venous; pulmonary

24. Neurohumoral activation and ventricular remodeling provide a _____ compensation to augment the _____ cardiac output and blood pressure seen in heart failure.
    A. temporary; increasing
    B. temporary; decreasing
    C. permanent; increasing
    D. permanent; decreasing

25. Neurohumoral activation involves all of the following *except:*
    A. parasympathetic stimulation.
    B. sympathetic stimulation.
    C. renin-angiotensin system.
    D. systemic hormones: vasopressin and atrial natriuretic peptide.

26. In ventricular remodeling, the _____ of the heart and the _____ of the ventricular wall are changed.
    A. valves; thickness
    B. valves; cellular composition
    C. shape; thickness
    D. shape; cellular composition

27. Pulmonary edema may develop under all of the following changes *except:*
    A. increased lymphatic drainage.
    B. increased pulmonary capillary pressure.
    C. increased capillary permeability.
    D. decreased blood oncotic pressure.

28. During inspiration, the alveoli expand and compress the blood vessels around them. This condition may lead to a(n):
    A. increased resistance to pulmonary blood flow.
    B. elevated pulmonary vascular resistance.
    C. increased pulmonary artery pressure.
    D. all of the above.

Questions 29 to 32: Ms. Downing, a 66-year-old patient diagnosed with congestive heart failure, is being treated for dyspnea on exertion. Her physician has ordered oxygen and bronchodilators via MDI.

29. Upon assessing Ms. Downing before therapy, you would expect to observe all of the following findings *except*:
    A. dyspnea.
    B. increased exercise tolerance.
    C. peripheral edema.
    D. fatigue and weakness.

30. Ms. Downing states that she has serious limitation while doing house chores and gardening at home after a few minutes. But she claims that "everything is fine after sitting down and resting for a few minutes." Her condition may be classified as Class _____ functional limitation.
    A. I
    B. II
    C. III
    D. IV

31. In reviewing Ms. Downing's medical records, which of the following is the *least* likely finding?
    A. Absence of S_3 and S_4 heart sounds
    B. Enlargement of the liver
    C. Swelling of the ankles and knees
    D. Bilateral crackles and wheezes

32. Since Ms. Downing's condition is chronic in nature, the most consistent radiographic finding would be:
    A. tension pneumothorax.
    B. cardiomegaly.
    C. atelectasis.
    D. pleural effusion.

Questions 33 to 38: Match the cardiac measurement and monitoring techniques in Column I with the respective characteristics or uses in Column II. Use each answer ONCE.

Column I

33. Electrocardiography
34. Echocardiography
35. Exercise stress testing
36. Radionucleotide imaging
37. Coronary angiography
38. Hemodynamic monitoring

Column II

A. Assessment of extent and severity of CAD; assessment of cardiac pump function; diagnosis of valvular disease
B. Imaging of myocardial perfusion with a radioisotope; assessment of valvular function, ejection fraction, and overall left ventricular size
C. Diagnosis of cardiac ischemia resulting from CAD under conditions of increased metabolic demand
D. Electrical conduction of the heart; assessment of rate, rhythm, and location of abnormal conduction
E. Placement of a catheter in pulmonary artery; measurement of preload, afterload, cardiac output, and mixed venous saturation
F. Diagnosis of valvular and myocardial diseases; screening test for CAD

39. In congestive heart failure, vasodilators may be beneficial to increase a patient's:
    A. cardiac output.
    B. preload as a result of venodilation.
    C. afterload as a result of arterial vasodilation.
    D. systemic and pulmonary blood pressure.

40. Hydralazine is an effective _____ and it may be used along with isosorbide dinitrate, _____.
    A. venodilator; also a venodilator
    B. venodilator; an arterial vasodilator at low doses
    C. arterial vasodilator; also an arterial vasodilator
    D. arterial vasodilator; a venodilator at low doses

41. _____ is recommended for all patients with left ventricular dysfunction _____ symptoms.
    A. Angiotensin-converting enzyme (ACE) inhibitors; regardless of
    B. Angiotensin-converting enzyme (ACE) inhibitors; with moderate to severe
    C. Calcium channel blockers; regardless of
    D. Calcium channel blockers; with moderate to severe

42. In congestive heart failure, diuretics may be beneficial to reduce:
    A. circulatory congestion.
    B. filling pressure.
    C. fluid retention.
    D. all of the above.

43. Digitalis has a positive _____ effect and it should be used with caution in patients with renal failure because of _____ drug clearance.
    A. chronotropic; reduced
    B. chronotropic; increased
    C. inotropic; reduced
    D. inotropic; increased

44. Theophylline, dobutamine, and dopamine are:
    A. inotropic agents.
    B. chronotropic agents.
    C. ß-blockers.
    D. vasodilators.

45. ß-blockers may be used to control symptoms of _____ heart failure by _____ the heart rate and providing sufficient time for ventricular filling.
    A. systolic; increasing
    B. systolic; decreasing
    C. diastolic; increasing
    D. diastolic; decreasing

46. Amiodarone is an _____ well-tolerated by patients with severe left ventricular dysfunction since it has the least _____ effect among drugs in this class.
    A. antiarrhythmic; positive inotropic
    B. antiarrhythmic; negative inotropic
    C. anticoagulant; bronchoconstrictive
    D. anticoagulant; vasoconstrictive

47. IABP, (intraaortic balloon pump), VADs (ventricular assist devices), and AICDs (automatic implantable cardioverter defibrillators) are _____ for cardiac failure.
    A. tailored therapies
    B. surgical treatments
    C. mechanical treatments
    D. noninvasive therapies

48. Which of the following is not a surgical treatment for cardiac failure?
    A. Cardioversion
    B. Cardiomyoplasty
    C. Heart transplantation
    D. Coronary revascularization

49. _____ is the recommended induction agent for intubation of patients with cardiovascular instability.
    A. Etomidate
    B. Propofol
    C. Opiate
    D. Benzodiazepine

50. For patients with cardiac failure, a tidal volume from _____ mL/kg should be used during mechanical ventilation.
    A. 5 to 7
    B. 8 to 10
    C. 11 to 12
    D. 12 to 14

51. Positive end-expiratory pressure (PEEP) increases the:
    A. intrathoracic pressure.
    B. afterload on the left ventricle.
    C. coronary perfusion.
    D. alveolar opening pressure.

CHAPTER 55

Chest Trauma

1. Knife and gunshot wounds to the thorax are examples of:
   A. blunt chest trauma.
   B. penetrating chest trauma.
   C. blood vessel trauma.
   D. pleural trauma.

2. What is the correct sequence for initial treatment of penetrating and blunt trauma?
   - I. Airway
   - II. Breathing
   - III. Circulation
   A. I and II
   B. I and III
   C. I, II, and III
   D. II and III

3. In blunt chest trauma, the most common injury involves:
   A. spleen rupture.
   B. shock.
   C. liver laceration.
   D. rib fracture.

Questions 4 to 8: Mr. Hightower, a patient in the emergency room, has a preliminary diagnosis of flail chest resulting from a motor vehicle accident.

4. On Mr. Hightower's chest radiograph, you would expect to see _____ rib fracture(s) in _____ place(s).
   A. one; a single
   B. two or more; a single
   C. one; two or more
   D. two; two or more

5. Mr. Hightower's chest radiograph confirms presence of flail chest. Based on this information, you would expect all of the following findings *except:*
   A. hyperinflation of lung.
   B. retention of secretions.
   C. increase work of breathing.
   D. rapid, shallow breathing.

6. As you are setting up the oxygen for Mr. Hightower, you notice that his breathing pattern is irregular and the rise of his chest does not correspond with inspiration. You would alert Dr. Freeman, the trauma physician, that Mr. Hightower has developed:
   A. apnea.
   B. hypoventilation.
   C. paradoxical breathing.
   D. Biot's respiration.

7. Dr. Freeman evaluates the chest radiograph and tells you that Mr. Hightower has developed hemothorax as well. This condition is:
   A. lung contusion.
   B. blood in the pleural space.
   C. air in the pleural space.
   D. pus in the pleural space.

8. Since the hemothorax is over 20% of the lung volume, Dr. Freeman decides to correct this problem by performing a(n) _____ before admitting the patient to the surgical unit.
   A. oral intubation
   B. blood transfusion
   C. needle biopsy
   D. tube thoracostomy

Questions 9 to 11: Match the treatments for pneumothorax or hemothorax in Column I with the common techniques in Column II. Use each answer ONCE.

Column I   Column II

9. Needle and syringe for emergency decompression of pneumothorax

10. Chest tube for pneumothorax

11. Chest tube for hemothorax

A. Insertion of a chest tube (20 to 22 French) into the third intercostal space along the midaxillary line

B. Insertion point in the midclavicular line into the third intercostal space

C. Insertion of a chest tube (38 to 40 French) into the fifth to sixth intercostal space along the midaxillary line

12. _____ is a major complication of providing analgesics to patients recovering from chest trauma.
    A. Excessive coughing
    B. Respiratory depression
    C. Immobility
    D. Hyperventilation

13. PCA is a method of pain control by:
    A. placing an intercostal catheter to the local site.
    B. administering the drug above the dura (epidural).
    C. using an intravenous route.
    D. allowing the patient to deliver the drug.

Question 14 to 18: Mr. Hightower, a patient admitted to the surgical unit by Dr. Freeman, is recovering from thoracic surgery. He is breathing spontaneously on 50% oxygen via face mask.

14. Dr. Freeman asks you to develop a care plan for Mr. Hightower. You would include in the care plan:
    A. coughing and deep breathing.
    B. bed rest.
    C. chest percussion.
    D. rib belt during coughing and deep breathing.

15. Mr. Hightower's ventilatory status is deteriorating and Dr. Freeman is considering reintubation. You would like to suggest mask CPAP (continuous positive airway pressure). Before you talk with Dr. Freeman about your suggestion, you would assess the patient for all of the following indications *except*:
    A. PaO_2/F_IO_2 between 100 and 250.
    B. patient is able to protect upper airway from aspiration.
    C. $PaCO_2$ at least 50 mm Hg.
    D. patient is alert and understands directions.

16. Dr. Freeman agrees to a CPAP trial. You would start the CPAP level at _____ cm H_2O and titrate it until the SpO_2 is above _____.
    A. 5; 92%
    B. 5; 98%
    C. 10; 92%
    D. 10; 98%

17. During the next hour, the CPAP level has reached 16 cm H_2O and Mr. Hightower's spontaneous respiratory rate has changed from 14/min to 26/min. His SpO_2 level has been at or below 90% on an F_IO_2 of 50% over this one-hour period. You would call Dr. Freeman and suggest:
    A. more pain control.
    B. intubation and mechanical ventilation.
    C. F_IO_2 to 100%.
    D. CPAP to 20 cm H_2O.

18. In addition to your suggestions in the previous question, you would recommend all of the following strategies *except*:
    A. PC-SIMV mode.
    B. keep plateau pressure below 10 cm H_2O.
    C. titrate PEEP to maintain SpO_2 over 60%.
    D. titrate PEEP to keep F_IO_2 below 60%.

19. Independent lung ventilation is used to:
    A. augment prone positioning of the patient.
    B. minimize use of PEEP.
    C. increase plateau pressure.
    D. ventilate patients with severe unilateral lung injury.

20. Cardiac tamponade is a complication of _____ chest trauma and it may exhibit _____.
    A. blunt; Beck's sign
    B. blunt; Beck's triad.
    C. penetrating; Beck's sign
    D. penetrating; Beck's triad.

21. In Case Study 2 of this chapter, the patient has a left lung compliance of 58 mL/cm H_2O and a right lung compliance of 32 mL/cm H_2O. This information implies that the patient's:
    A. left lung is affected by the chest trauma more than the right lung.
    B. lungs are affected equally.
    C. right lung is affected by the chest trauma more than the left lung.
    D. Insufficient information to determine answer

CHAPTER 56

Burn and Inhalation Injuries

1. During the first phase of wound care, the main purpose is to:
   A. close small, complex wounds.
   B. evaluate and provide accurate fluid resuscitation.
   C. identify all full-thickness wounds.
   D. maintain range of motion.

2. Massive capillary leak occurs during the _____ phase of wound care.
   A. first
   B. second
   C. third
   D. fourth

3. The preferred method to determine the extent of a burn injury is the:
   A. rule of nines.
   B. palmar surface of the hand.
   C. Lund-Browder chart.
   D. scar index.

4. Third-degree burn causes:
   A. wounds that involve subcutaneous tissue, tendon, or bone.
   B. red, wet, very painful wounds.
   C. leathery, dry, insensate, waxy wounds.
   D. red, dry, painful wounds.

5. Fluid resuscitation is necessary in severe burns because of:
   A. dehydration.
   B. evaporation.
   C. diuresis.
   D. diffuse capillary leakage.

6. Circumferential burn wounds of the torso hinder ventilation due to:
   A. increased chest wall compliance.
   B. swelling of tissue beneath the inelastic eschar.
   C. swelling of large airways.
   D. carbon monoxide poisoning.

7. The purpose of escharotomy is to:
   A. reduce infection.
   B. facilitate wound healing.
   C. improve ventilation.
   D. ease pain.

8. The treatment for inhalation injury typically consists of:
   A. artificial airway and mechanical ventilation.
   B. hyperbaric oxygenation.
   C. established protocol.
   D. supportive therapies depending on needs.

9. Inhalation injury may lead to all of the following *except:*
   A. increased compliance.
   B. increased airflow resistance.
   C. pneumonia.
   D. alveolar flooding.

10. Presence of carbonaceous debris in the mouth or sputum, singed nasal hairs, and facial burns are signs of:
    A. smoke inhalation.
    B. circumferential burn wounds.
    C. carbon monoxide poisoning.
    D. inhalation injury.

11. _____ is the gold standard for diagnosis of inhalation injury.
    A. Carboxyhemoglobin level
    B. Bronchoscopy
    C. Lung scan
    D. Lung biopsy

Questions 12 to 16. Match the management strategies of inhalation injury in Column I with the respective rationales in Column II. Use each answer ONCE.

Column I

Column II

12. Bronchodilators

13. Endotracheal tube

14. Focused antibiotics

15. Mechanical ventilation

16. Chest physiotherapy

A. To treat infection
B. To support respiratory failure
C. To relieve upper airway obstruction
D. To treat small airway obstruction
E. To treat bronchospasm

17. Infection usually occurs toward the end of the _____ postinjury week and it should be treated with antibiotics based on information from sputum _____.
    A. first; culture
    B. first; gram stain
    C. second; culture
    D. second; gram stain

Questions 18 to 20: Mr. Queen, a patient who has been rescued from a house fire, suffers from inhalation injury. While in the emergency room, his SpO$_2$ reading on room air is 99% on 2 L/min of oxygen via nasal cannula. He is breathing spontaneously and no cyanosis is noted.

18. Based on this information, you would:
    A. discontinue the oxygen.
    B. change oxygen to 28% via Venturi mask.
    C. change oxygen to 40% via aerosol mask.
    D. change oxygen to non-rebreathing mask at 15 L/min.

19. Your decision is based on the inaccuracy of the _____ under this patient condition.
    A. pulse oximeter reading
    B. oxygen concentration
    C. low flow characteristic of nasal cannula
    D. oxygen flow meter

20. High concentration of _____ is the treatment for carbon monoxide inhalation because the half-life of carboxyhemoglobin (COHb) under this treatment modality is slightly over _____ hour.
    A. nitrogen; one
    B. nitrogen; five
    C. oxygen; one
    D. oxygen; five

CHAPTER 57

Neuromuscular Dysfunction

1. In neuromuscular dysfunction, the respiratory pump may be impaired at the level of the:
   A. central nervous system and spinal cord.
   B. peripheral nerve and neuromuscular junction.
   C. inspiratory and expiratory muscles.
   D. all of the above.

Questions 2 to 5: Match the levels of pathologic injury in Column I with the respective neuromuscular diseases in Column II. Use each answer ONCE.

Column I

Column II

2. Upper motor neuron—cerebral spinal cord

3. Lower motor neuron—anterior horn cells

4. Lower motor neuron—peripheral nerves

5. Lower motor neuron—neuromuscular junction

A. Myasthenia gravis, botulism
B. Stroke, trauma
C. Phrenic nerve injury, diabetes mellitus, Guillain-Barré syndrome (GBS)
D. Poliomyelitis, amyotrophic lateral sclerosis

6. The pathophysiology of respiratory failure in patients with neuromuscular disease typically shows:
   A. decreased $PaCO_2$.
   B. increased lung volumes.
   C. increased PaO_2.
   D. hypoventilation.

7. _____ is an accurate test of a patient's central respiratory drive that is independent of underlying respiratory mechanics.
   A. Pulmonary function
   B. Mouth occlusion pressure
   C. Peak flow
   D. Arterial blood gases

8. In patients with neuromuscular dysfunction, you would expect to find:
   A. increased lung volumes.
   B. increased lung compliance.
   C. rapid, shallow breathing pattern.
   D. hyperinflation.

9. During the _____ stage of neuromuscular disease, _____ are common findings.
   A. early; alkalosis and hypocapnia
   B. early; hypoxemia and hypercapnia
   C. late; alkalosis and hypocapnia
   D. late; hypoxemia and hypercapnia

10. Rapid, shallow breathing during REM sleep is undesirable because it leads to:
    A. increased dead space ventilation.
    B. increased intrapulmonary shunt.
    C. decreased dead space ventilation.
    D. decreased intrapulmonary shunt.

11. Aspiration, stridor, obstructive sleep apnea, and hypopnea are signs of:
    A. loss of gag reflex.
    B. restrictive lung disease.
    C. upper airway dysfunction.
    D. lower motor neuron lesion.

12. An acute ascending paralysis of the lower extremities may suggest:
    A. GBS.
    B. myasthenia gravis.
    C. poliomyelitis.
    D. multiple sclerosis.

13. In evaluating a patient's clinical history, the common symptoms of respiratory muscle weakness include all of the following *except*:
    A. dyspnea on exertion.
    B. increased peak expiratory flow.
    C. inability to clear secretions and weak cough.
    D. frequent respiratory tract infection.

Questions 14 to 17: *Ms. Garland, a 66-year-old, 50-Kg patient in the neurology intensive care unit, has an admitting diagnosis of cerebrovascular accident (CVA). She is breathing spontaneously on 5 L/min of oxygen via nasal cannula.*

14. Ms. Garland's physical examination might show:
    A. use of accessory muscles.
    B. tachypnea.
    C. paradoxical breathing pattern.
    D. all of the above.

15. Her blood gases on room air prior to admission would most likely show hypoxemia due to:
    I. Atelectasis
    II. V/Q mismatch
    III. Shunt
    IV. Retained secretions
    A. I, II, and III
    B. I, III, and IV
    C. II and IV
    D. All of the above

16. Over the past three hours since admission to the unit, Ms. Garland's hourly FVC measurements show: 1.7 L, 1.8 L, 1.7 L. You would suggest to her physician:
    A. continue with hourly FVC.
    B. intubate immediately.
    C. intubate and provide mechanical ventilation.
    D. perform tracheotomy.

17. Ms. Garland's chest radiograph on admission would most likely show:
    A. pleural effusion.
    B. unilateral elevated hemidiaphragm.
    C. loss of lung volume.
    D. hyperinflation.

Questions 18 to 21: *Match the techniques of respiratory muscle function assessment in Column I with the respective descriptions in Column II. Use each answer ONCE.*

Column I

18. Maximum mouth pressure

19. Forced vital capacity

20. Maximum voluntary ventilation

21. Transdiaphragmatic pressure measurement

Column II

A. To assess respiratory muscle endurance
B. To measure diaphragm strength
C. To assess respiratory muscle dysfunction in the absence of symptoms
D. To predict impending respiratory failure

22. _____ stroke often results in aspiration and Cheyne-Stokes breathing.
    A. Parkinson's
    B. Spinal cord
    C. Hemispheric
    D. Brainstem

23. In patients with _____ cervical cord injury, adequate spontaneous breathing is impossible. This is because at this level all major respiratory muscles, including the diaphragm, are paralyzed.
    A. C1 to C3
    B. C3 to C5
    C. C5 to C6
    D. below C6

24. In patients with low cervical cord injury, all of the following are often observed with the *exception* of:
    A. retention of secretions.
    B. hyperinflation.
    C. atelectasis.
    D. pneumonia.

25. Parkinson's disease:
    A. is caused by aging.
    B. rarely causes lung infection.
    C. produces obstructive and restrictive disease patterns.
    D. produces increased flow rates.

26. Multiple sclerosis:
    A. causes paralysis of the diaphragm.
    B. is a disease of the autonomic nervous system.
    C. does not affect automatic respiration.
    D. may lead to central sleep apnea.

27. Amyotrophic lateral sclerosis is a _____ disorder of the _____ motor neurons.
    A. neurodegenerative; upper
    B. neurodegenerative; upper and lower
    C. paralytic; upper
    D. paralytic; upper and lower

28. In patients with amyotrophic lateral sclerosis, the reduction in _____ is _____.
    A. tidal volume; gradual
    B. tidal volume; sudden
    C. vital capacity and mouth pressures; gradual
    D. vital capacity and mouth pressures; sudden

29. Noninvasive positive pressure ventilation is beneficial for many patients with:
    A. poliomyelitis.
    B. postpoliomyelitis dystrophy.
    C. amyotrophic lateral sclerosis.
    D. all of the above.

30. Phrenic nerve injury:
    A. produces bilateral diaphragm paralysis.
    B. increases dyspnea in supine position.
    C. is treated with fluoroscopy.
    D. all of the above.

Questions 31 to 36: Ms. Rowland, a patient with a preliminary diagnosis of GBS, is in the intensive care unit for "respiratory failure." She is 40 years old, 5'3" and 110 lbs (50 Kg).

31. Ms. Rowland's preliminary diagnosis may be confirmed by examining the:
    A. chest radiograph.
    B. cerebrospinal fluid.
    C. blood gas results.
    D. pulmonary function results.

32. _____ would be diagnostic of GBS.
    A. Bilateral infiltrates on chest radiograph
    B. Increased protein content with few cells in spinal fluid
    C. Acute respiratory acidosis with severe hypoxemia
    D. Obstructive and restrictive lung functions

33. A nursing student asks you about this syndrome. You would explain to him that GBS is a(n) _____ idiopathic polyneuritis typically presenting as a(n) _____ symmetric paralysis of the lower extremities.
    A. acute; ascending
    B. acute; descending
    C. chronic; ascending
    D. chronic; descending

34. Her physician asks you to evaluate Ms. Rowland for the progression of the GBS. You would perform:
    A. stat vital capacity measurement.
    B. serial vital capacity measurements.
    C. stat peak flow measurement.
    D. serial peak flow measurements.

35. Three hours following admission to the ICU, Ms. Rowland's vital capacity (VC) is 800 mL. You would call the physician and recommend:
    A. oral intubation.
    B. nasal intubation.
    C. intubation and mechanical ventilation.
    D. intubation and 60% oxygen via continuous heated aerosol.

36. In addition to the previous recommendation, you would suggest to the physician that aggressive pulmonary toilet be done to prevent _____.
    A. stridor.
    B. pneumothorax.
    C. pleural effusion.
    D. atelectasis.

37. _____ is an autoimmune disorder that impairs the transmission of neural impulses across the neuromuscular junction.
    A. Myasthenia gravis
    B. GBS
    C. Critical illness polyneuropathy
    D. Botulism

38. One of the reasons for myasthenic crisis to occur is _____ and this can be verified with _____ testing.
    A. excessive anticholinergic medications; Tensilon
    B. excessive acetylcholine; cholinesterase
    C. insufficient anticholinergic medications; Tensilon
    D. insufficient acetylcholine; cholinesterase

39. The first line of treatment for myasthenia gravis is:
    A. cholinesterase agents.
    B. anticholinesterase agents.
    C. mechanical ventilation.
    D. low-dose corticosteroids.

40. Mr. Taylor, a patient in the emergency department, complained of gastrointestinal symptoms a few days ago after opening and eating some food from an "old and rusty" can. He states mild to moderate paralysis of the neck, body, and extremities in the last 12 hours. Mr. Taylor is likely suffering from:
    A. botulism.
    B. acid maltase deficiency or systemic lupus erythematosus.
    C. chronic steroid myopathy or Eaton-Lambert syndrome.
    D. Duchenne muscular dystrophy or myotonic dystrophy.

41. Treatment of neuromuscular dysfunction includes:
    A. assisted coughing.
    B. frog breathing.
    C. noninvasive positive-pressure ventilation.
    D. all of the above.

42. In patients with neuromuscular dysfunction, noninvasive positive-pressure ventilation should be considered when:
    A. airway control is inadequate.
    B. secretions are thick and copious.
    C. hemodynamic status is stable.
    D. all of the above.

43. Negative pressure ventilation:
    A. does not require an artificial airway.
    B. is easy to set up and maintain.
    C. may be used to treat obstructive sleep apnea.
    D. facilitates nursing care.

44. The widespread use of diaphragmatic pacing is limited due to:
    A. high cost.
    B. potential for sudden failure.
    C. induction of diaphragmatic fatigue.
    D. all of the above.

CHAPTER 58

Management of Obstructive Sleep Apnea Syndrome

1. Weight gain is the most important etiologic factor in the development of:
   A. central apnea.
   B. obstructive sleep apnea.
   C. mixed apnea.
   D. hypoventilation.

2. Sleep apnea is defined by a(n):
   A. apnea count of at least 5/hour.
   B. apnea/hypopnea index of at least 5/hour.
   C. apnea count of at least 15/hour.
   D. apnea/hypopnea index of at least 15/hour.

3. When obstructive sleep apnea is caused by weight gain, solutions may include all of the following *except*:
   A. gastric reduction.
   B. pharmacologic agents.
   C. bowel bypass surgery.
   D. exercise.

4. In obstructive sleep apnea, the initial treatment of choice is:
   A. oxygen therapy.
   B. pharmacologic agents.
   C. nasal CPAP.
   D. mechanical ventilation.

5. The hindrance to nasal CPAP therapy is:
   A. poor patient compliance.
   B. high cost.
   C. complicated setup.
   D. all of the above.

6. The optimal nasal CPAP level should be:
   A. at least 10 cm H_2O.
   B. at least 15 cm H_2O.
   C. based on arterial blood gas results.
   D. determined by an attended polysomnogram.

7. Side effects related to nasal CPAP include all of the following *except*:
   A. nasal dryness, congestion, or drip.
   B. claustrophobia.
   C. hyperventilation.
   D. aerophagia.

8. Oral appliances:
   A. include tongue retaining and mandibular advancing devices.
   B. constrict the pharyngeal cross-sectional area.
   C. are effective for most patients with obstructive sleep apnea.
   D. reduce pain at the temporomandibular joint.

9. Dental examination is required prior to:
   A. titration of CPAP level.
   B. fitting of oral appliance.
   C. oropharyngeal surgery.
   D. use of oronasal mask.

10. Side effects related to oral appliances include all of the following *except*:
    A. TMJ discomfort.
    B. dry mouth.
    C. lack of salivation.
    D. jaw and teeth discomfort.

11. Oropharyngeal surgery:
    A. includes uvulopalatopharyngoplasty and laser-assisted uvulopalatoplasty.
    B. has a success rate of about 75%.
    C. should not be done with other interventions such as tonsillectomy.
    D. all of the above.

CHAPTER 59

Lung Cancer

1. _____ lung cancer accounts for _____ deaths annually worldwide.
   A. Benign; 100,000
   B. Benign; 1,000,000
   C. Malignant; 100,000
   D. Malignant; 1,000,000

2. Tobacco smoking is the primary cause of _____ lung cancer and this type of cancer spreads _____.
   A. small cell; slowly
   B. small cell; quickly
   C. non-small cell; slowly
   D. non-small cell; quickly

3. The major difference between lung cancer and other cancers is that lung cancer is largely:
   A. related to family history.
   B. related to genetics.
   C. preventable.
   D. treatable.

4. The relative risk of lung cancer is linked to all of the following factors *except*:
   A. occupational exposure to carcinogens.
   B. exposure to secondhand smoke.
   C. number of cigarettes smoked per day.
   D. number of children.

5. In patients diagnosed with lung cancer, which of the following signs and symptoms is *least* likely an initial presentation?
   A. Digital clubbing
   B. Hemoptysis
   C. Cough
   D. Chest pain

Questions 6 to 10: Match the presentations of lung cancer in Column I with the respective descriptions in Column II. Use each answer ONCE.

Column I

6. Dyspnea
7. Hemoptysis
8. Chest pain
9. Dysphagia
10. Extrathoracic pain

Column II

A. Compression of the esophagus due to local spread of proximal tumors or lymph node masses
B. Hematogenous spread of the cancer to the central nervous system, bone, liver, and adrenal glands
C. Characteristic of bleeding tumors
D. Result of airway obstruction with atelectasis, postobstructive pneumonitis, and other conditions that affect gas exchange
E. Extension of a peripheral mass to the pleura or the chest wall

11. Solitary pulmonary nodule is:
    A. invisible on routine chest radiograph.
    B. usually symptomatic.
    C. the most curable presentation of bronchogenic cancer.
    D. caused by cigarette smoking in majority of cases.

12. Benign and malignant solitary pulmonary nodules may be differentiated based on all of the following criteria *except*:
    A. clinical criteria (e.g., age, symptoms, history).
    B. radiographic criteria (e.g., size, location, and doubling time of nodule).
    C. computed tomography criteria (e.g., patterns of calcification).
    D. pulmonary function criteria (e.g., diffusing capacity, closing volume).

Questions 13 to 17. Match the diagnostic techniques for lung cancer in Column I with the respective application in Column II. Use each answer ONCE.

Column I

13. Sputum tests

14. Bronchoscopy

15. Mediastinoscopy

16. Transbronchial needle aspiration

17. Pleural biopsy

Column II

A. For work-up of central and mediastinal lesions

B. For central lung mass on chest radiograph

C. For lesions close to the tracheobronchial tree

D. For malignant effusion

E. For patients with mediastinal lymphadenopathy

18. TNM refers to:
   A. primary tumor, local lymph nodes, proximal metastasis.
   B. primary tumor, regional lymph nodes, distant metastasis.
   C. secondary tumor, local lymph nodes, proximal metastasis.
   D. secondary tumor, regional lymph nodes, distant metastasis.

19. Knowledge of the staging system for lung cancer can help to determine the:
   A. appropriate treatments.
   B. cost of medical care.
   C. necessary work-up.
   D. prognosis.

20. Pulmonary function testing is recommended for patients:
   A. with malignant lung cancer.
   B. with benign lung cancer.
   C. who are symptomatic during initial exam.
   D. who are candidates for surgery.

21. Traditional treatment of lung cancer includes all of the following *except:*
   A. smoking cessation.
   B. surgery.
   C. radiotherapy.
   D. chemotherapy.

22. Small cell lung cancer:
   A. has a low mortality rate if left untreated.
   B. has a high relapse rate with chemotherapy.
   C. may be treated with medication.
   D. has good results with surgical intervention.

23. For _____ stage non-small cell lung cancer, _____ is the treatment of choice.
   A. early; surgery
   B. early; chemotherapy
   C. late; surgery
   D. late; chemotherapy

24. Neutropenia, mucositis, infection, neurologic toxicity are some complications of:
   A. radiotherapy.
   B. chemotherapeutic drugs.
   C. surgery.
   D. biopsy.

25. Mediastinal fibrosis, constrictive pericarditis, restrictive cardiomyopathy, and accelerated coronary artery disease are some _____ complications of _____.
   A. acute; radiotherapy
   B. acute; chemotherapeutic drugs
   C. chronic; radiotherapy
   D. chronic; chemotherapeutic drugs

26. The _____ is used to assess a patient's performance as a percentage of normal activities.
   A. Karnofsky Performance Scale
   B. resectability
   C. tumor differentiation
   D. histologic subtype

27. Many lung cancers can be prevented by:
   A. smoking cessation.
   B. screening for lung cancer.
   C. interventions to prevent disease progression.
   D. all of the above.

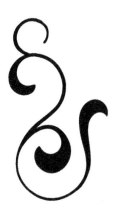

Answer Key to Self-Assessment Questions

Chapter 1—History of the Respiratory Care Profession
1. B
2. D
3. A
4. C
5. B
6. A
7. D
8. C
9. B
10. C
11. D
12. B
13. A
14. D
15. D
16. C

Chapter 2— Professional Organizations
1. A
2. B
3. C
4. A
5. C
6. D
7. C
8. D
9. B
10. A
11. D
12. B
13. B
14. C
15. E
16. C
17. B
18. A
19. D
20. A

Chapter 3—Health Care Trends and Evolving Roles of Respiratory Care Professionals
1. D
2. A
3. B
4. C
5. B
6. D
7. C
8. A
9. D
10. D
11. B
12. B
13. A
14. D
15. C
16. A
17. B
18. C
19. A
20. C
21. A
22. C

Chapter 4—Critical Thinking and Problem-Based Learning in Respiratory Care
1. D
2. D
3. B
4. D
5. A
6. B
7. C
8. A
9. D
10. D
11. B
12. C
13. B
14. B
15. A
16. B
17. D
18. B
19. A
20. A
21. D

Chapter 5—Ethics of Health Care Delivery
1. D
2. C
3. A
4. A
5. C
6. B
7. A
8. B
9. C
10. D
11. E
12. G
13. A
14. F
15. D
16. C
17. B
18. C
19. B
20. D
21. A
22. D
23. A
24. C
25. B
26. D
27. A
28. B
29. A
30. D

Chapter 6— Communication Skills
1. D
2. D
3. B
4. A
5. E
6. C
7. C
8. E
9. A
10. B
11. D
12. A
13. C
14. B
15. D
16. C
17. A
18. E
19. A
20. D
21. B
22. F
23. C
24. D
25. A
26. B
27. C
28. C
29. B
30. A
31. C

32. A
33. B
34. A
35. B
36. C
37. C
38. A
39. D
40. B
41. B

Chapter 7—Decision Making and the Role of the Consultant
1. C
2. D
3. B
4. A
5. B
6. B
7. A
8. D
9. C
10. A
11. B
12. C
13. A
14. D
15. B
16. C
17. C
18. A
19. D
20. C
21. A
22. B
23. B
24. D
25. D
26. A
27. D
28. C

Chapter 8—Patient Education
1. C
2. C
3. D
4. B
5. D
6. A
7. C
8. D
9. B
10. A
11. B

12. A
13. D
14. C
15. A
16. B
17. D
18. B
19. C
20. B

Chapter 9—Documentation and Medical Information Management
1. A
2. C
3. B
4. A
5. D
6. D
7. C
8. D
9. A
10. B
11. C
12. B
13. A
14. B
15. C
16. B
17. D
18. A
19. B

Chapter 10—Assessing Outcomes
1. B
2. A
3. B
4. B
5. A
6. D
7. D
8. A
9. B
10. D
11. B
12. A
13. A
14. B
15. C
16. D
17. C
18. A
19. B
20. D

21. D

Chapter 11—Health Care Reimbursement
1. C
2. D
3. B
4. A
5. B
6. C
7. D
8. A
9. B
10. C
11. D
12. B
13. B
14. C
15. A
16. E
17. D
18. A
19. B
20. A
21. E
22. D
23. A
24. C
25. D
26. C
27. A
28. B
29. D
30. A
31. A
32. C
33. B
34. B
35. B
36. D

Chapter 12—Evaluating and Accessing Medical Information
1. C
2. D
3. D
4. D
5. D
6. A
7. E
8. C
9. B
10. A
11. A

12. B
13. D
14. C
15. C
16. C
17. A
18. C
19. B
20. C
21. B
22. D
23. C
24. D
25. B
26. C
27. D
28. B
29. D
30. C

Chapter 13—Mathematical Aspects of Respiratory Care
1. E
2. A
3. B
4. D
5. A
6. C
7. A
8. F
9. B
10. G
11. D
12. E
13. A
14. E
15. D
16. A
17. F
18. C
19. B
20. C
21. A
22. D
23. B
24. A
25. C
26. A
27. D
28. F
29. D
30. A
31. C
32. B
33. D

34. D

Chapter 14—
Application of
Physical Principles

1. A
2. C
3. C
4. D
5. A
6. H
7. B
8. F
9. B
10. C
11. A
12. D
13. B
14. B
15. B
16. C
17. D
18. D
19. A
20. D
21. A
22. D
23. B
24. A
25. C
26. B
27. C
28. D
29. B
30. D

Chapter 15—
Chemistry for
Respiratory Care

1. A
2. B
3. D
4. C
5. B
6. A
7. D
8. D
9. C
10. D
11. B
12. B
13. D
14. A
15. B
16. B
17. A

18. B
19. B
20. D
21. C
22. A
23. C
24. C
25. B
26. C
27. A
28. D
29. B
30. C
31. A
32. A
33. D
34. C
35. B
36. C
37. A
38. B
39. A
40. D
41. C
42. B
43. B
44. C
45. B
46. C
47. A
48. A
49. A
50. D
51. A
52. C
53. B
54. A

Chapter 16—
Respiratory
Microbiology,
Infection, and
Infection Control

1. C
2. A
3. D
4. C
5. B
6. C
7. A
8. B
9. A
10. C
11. B
12. C
13. A

14. D
15. B
16. C
17. C
18. B
19. D
20. C
21. D
22. B
23. A
24. C
25. D
26. A
27. B
28. A
29. D
30. D

Chapter 17—
Cardiopulmonary
Anatomy and
Physiology

1. D
2. A
3. B
4. C
5. C
6. C
7. E
8. B
9. A
10. D
11. D
12. A
13. D
14. B
15. C
16. D
17. B
18. E
19. A
20. C
21. A
22. B
23. A
24. D
25. B
26. D
27. B
28. D
29. A
30. D
31. C
32. A
33. D
34. B

35. B
36. C
37. A
38. B
39. C
40. A
41. D
42. A
43. C

Chapter 18—
Respiratory
Pharmacology

1. A
2. C
3. B
4. B
5. D
6. D
7. D
8. C
9. A
10. B
11. A
12. C
13. D
14. B
15. C
16. A
17. A
18. C
19. B
20. B
21. C
22. D
23. A
24. C
25. D
26. A
27. B
28. C
29. C
30. A
31. C
32. D
33. F
34. D
35. G
36. B
37. A
38. E
39. C
40. A
41. B
42. A
43. C

44. D
45. B
46. D
47. C
48. B
49. C
50. B
51. D
52. A
53. C
54. D
55. E
56. D
57. A
58. B
59. C
60. A
61. B
62. E
63. A
64. D
65. C
66. B
67. A
68. D
69. B
70. D
71. A
72. A
73. C

Chapter 19—
History and Physical
Examination

1. C
2. D
3. B
4. D
5. B
6. C
7. B
8. C
9. D
10. A
11. E
12. A
13. D
14. C
15. B
16. A
17. C
18. B
19. A
20. D
21. C
22. A

23. D
24. A
25. C
26. D
27. B
28. D
29. B
30. A
31. B
32. C
33. A

Chapter 20—Blood
Chemistries and
Hematology

1. C
2. B
3. A
4. D
5. A
6. B
7. D
8. A
9. B
10. C
11. A
12. D
13. C
14. C
15. D
16. C
17. C
18. H
19. F
20. A
21. G
22. B
23. D
24. E
25. C
26. D
27. B
28. D
29. B
30. A
31. B
32. D
33. C
34. B
35. D
36. B
37. C
38. A
39. A
40. B
41. C

42. A
43. D

Chapter 21—Arterial
Blood Gases

1. D
2. B
3. B
4. A
5. D
6. C
7. A
8. A
9. B
10. C
11. A
12. C
13. C
14. A
15. B
16. B
17. D
18. B
19. A
20. D
21. D
22. C
23. B
24. B
25. C
26. A
27. D
28. E
29. B
30. C
31. D
32. A
33. C
34. A
35. B
36. A
37. F
38. C
39. D
40. D
41. C
42. B
43. A
44. C
45. A
46. B
47. D
48. B

Chapter 22—
Nutrition Assessment
and Support

1. B
2. C
3. A
4. A
5. B
6. D
7. C
8. D
9. C
10. D
11. A
12. B
13. C
14. B
15. D
16. A
17. C
18. C
19. B
20. B
21. D
22. A
23. D

Chapter 23—
Cardiac Assessment

1. D
2. C
3. B
4. A
5. C
6. C
7. D
8. B
9. A
10. C
11. D
12. C
13. D
14. A
15. B
16. B
17. C
18. A
19. D
20. A
21. D
22. B
23. C
24. A
25. D
26. C
27. A

28. D
29. C
30. C
31. A
32. B
33. B
34. A
35. D
36. A
37. D
38. B

Chapter 24—
Imaging the Thorax
1. C
2. A
3. A
4. C
5. C
6. B
7. B
8. D
9. D
10. A
11. C
12. D
13. A
14. B
15. D
16. B
17. C
18. A
19. D
20. C
21. A
22. B

Chapter 25—
Pulmonary
Function Testing
1. D
2. B
3. D
4. C
5. A
6. B
7. C
8. C
9. A
10. D
11. B
12. A
13. B
14. D
15. D
16. A

17. D
18. D
19. B
20. A
21. B
22. C
23. C
24. B
25. C
26. C
27. D
28. C
29. A
30. D

Chapter 26—
Hemodynamic and Gas
Exchange Monitoring
1. D
2. D
3. C
4. B
5. A
6. D
7. C
8. E
9. B
10. A
11. B
12. B
13. A
14. D
15. D
16. B
17. D
18. C
19. B
20. C
21. A
22. C
23. A
24. A
25. C
26. A
27. B
28. C
29. B
30. C
31. A
32. D

Chapter 27—
Exercise Assessment
1. A
2. D
3. C

4. A
5. B
6. B
7. D
8. C
9. C
10. A
11. B
12. A
13. A
14. C
15. D
16. B
17. D

Chapter 28—
Fiberoptic
Bronchoscopy
1. A
2. C
3. D
4. C
5. B
6. A
7. A
8. B
9. C
10. A
11. D
12. C
13. B
14. B
15. B
16. C
17. D
18. A
19. B
20. D
21. E
22. C
23. F
24. A
25. D
26. D

Chapter 29—
Sleep Assessment
1. C
2. A
3. D
4. C
5. C
6. D
7. D
8. C
9. A

10. F
11. E
12. D
13. B
14. B
15. D
16. B
17. A
18. B
19. A

Chapter 30—Infant
Apnea Monitoring
1. B
2. D
3. E
4. D
5. A
6. C
7. B
8. D
9. A
10. C
11. D
12. B
13. A
14. B
15. C
16. D
17. C
18. A
19. C
20. A

Chapter 31—Medical
Gases—Manufacture,
Storage, and Delivery
1. B
2. D
3. D
4. C
5. A
6. B
7. E
8. D
9. F
10. A
11. C
12. B
13. A
14. C
15. B
16. C
17. E
18. A
19. F

20. B
21. D
22. A
23. B
24. C
25. A
26. C
27. D
28. A
29. C
30. D
31. D

**Chapter 32—
Oxygen Therapy:
Administration and
Management**

1. B
2. D
3. B
4. A
5. B
6. A
7. C
8. B
9. C
10. C
11. D
12. B
13. A
14. D
15. D
16. C
17. C
18. C
19. D
20. A
21. A
22. B
23. D
24. A
25. C
26. D

**Chapter 33—
Hyperbaric Oxygen**

1. B
2. C
3. C
4. E
5. D
6. A
7. C
8. B
9. A
10. B

11. D
12. C
13. A
14. B
15. A
16. D
17. B
18. A
19. C
20. D
21. C
22. B
23. A
24. D

**Chapter 34—Humidity
and Aerosol Therapy**

1. D
2. B
3. D
4. D
5. D
6. A
7. C
8. B
9. A
10. B
11. C
12. C
13. B
14. A
15. D
16. C
17. C
18. B
19. A
20. B
21. A
22. D
23. C
24. B
25. D
26. C
27. C
28. B
29. D
30. C
31. A
32. A
33. A
34. B
35. C
36. D
37. A

**Chapter 35—Secretion
Clearance Techniques**

1. D
2. B
3. C
4. A
5. C
6. B
7. D
8. D
9. A
10. D
11. C
12. B
13. A
14. B
15. C
16. B
17. A
18. D
19. C
20. C
21. A
22. B
23. D
24. A

**Chapter 36—
Airway Management**

1. D
2. A
3. B
4. A
5. A
6. B
7. C
8. D
9. A
10. A
11. D
12. A
13. B
14. C
15. C
16. B
17. C
18. B
19. C
20. A
21. C
22. C
23. B
24. D
25. C
26. C
27. B

28. C
29. A
30. B
31. D
32. C
33. B
34. D
35. D
36. B
37. A
38. D
39. B
40. D

**Chapter 37—
Cardiopulmonary
Resuscitation**

1. D
2. C
3. A
4. A
5. C
6. D
7. D
8. D
9. B
10. A
11. B
12. D
13. C
14. B
15. B
16. A
17. A
18. C
19. B
20. C
21. C
22. D
23. E
24. B
25. A

**Chapter 38—
Pulmonary
Rehabilitation**

1. A
2. B
3. C
4. A
5. B
6. D
7. B
8. B
9. D
10. B

11. A
12. B
13. C
14. A
15. B
16. C
17. A
18. C
19. A
20. D
21. A
22. C
23. A
24. A
25. C

Chapter 39—
Mechanical
Ventilators:
Classification and
Principles of Operation
1. C
2. D
3. C
4. C
5. B
6. B
7. D
8. C
9. C
10. B
11. B
12. D
13. D
14. B
15. A
16. A
17. B
18. C
19. D
20. B
21. B
22. C
23. A
24. D
25. C
26. C
27. D
28. A
29. B
30. E
31. B
32. A
33. D
34. D
35. B

36. C
37. D
38. D
39. B
40. D
41. A
42. E
43. A
44. C
45. B

Chapter 40—
Mechanical Ventilation
1. D
2. A
3. B
4. D
5. A
6. F
7. C
8. E
9. B
10. D
11. A
12. C
13. D
14. C
15. B
16. A
17. C
18. B
19. A
20. B
21. A
22. D
23. B
24. A
25. C
26. B
27. D
28. C
29. B
30. C

Chapter 41—Neonatal
Mechanical Ventilation
1. A
2. D
3. B
4. C
5. C
6. A
7. A
8. D
9. C
10. A

11. B
12. B
13. C
14. A
15. B
16. C
17. B
18. B
19. D
20. D
21. C
22. C
23. D
24. B
25. A
26. A
27. D
28. C
29. A
30. B
31. B
32. D
33. B
34. A
35. A
36. C
37. D
38. C
39. D
40. B
41. C
42. D

Chapter 42—
Mechanical Ventilation
in Alternate Care Sites
1. D
2. C
3. B
4. A
5. C
6. C
7. B
8. A
9. B
10. A
11. D
12. B
13. C
14. A
15. D
16. B
17. C
18. B
19. C
20. B

21. A
22. C
23. D
24. A
25. D

Chapter 43—
Noninvasive
Ventilation and
Continuous Positive
Airway Pressure
1. D
2. C
3. A
4. B
5. D
6. B
7. C
8. A
9. B
10. C
11. D
12. A
13. C
14. D
15. B
16. C
17. A
18. D
19. D
20. A
21. B

Chapter 44—
Nonconventional
Respiratory
Therapeutics
1. B
2. A
3. C
4. D
5. A
6. A
7. B
8. A
9. D
10. C
11. B
12. A
13. C
14. B
15. D
16. D
17. C

Chapter 45—
Principles of Disease
Management
1. A
2. D
3. C
4. D
5. B
6. B
7. A
8. C
9. B
10. B
11. D
12. E
13. A
14. C
15. A
16. C
17. D
18. A

Chapter 46—Asthma
1. B
2. D
3. A
4. B
5. D
6. A
7. C
8. A
9. B
10. C
11. C
12. D
13. C
14. A
15. B
16. E
17. D
18. A
19. C
20. D
21. C
22. A
23. C
24. B
25. A
26. D
27. B
28. C
29. B
30. A
31. D
32. B

Chapter 47—
Chronic Obstructive
Pulmonary Disease
1. A
2. B
3. A
4. C
5. C
6. D
7. C
8. B
9. A
10. B
11. A
12. A
13. B
14. A
15. C
16. C
17. A
18. D
19. A
20. B
21. D
22. A
23. D
24. B
25. C
26. A
27. B
28. D
29. C
30. A
31. B
32. D
33. C
34. D
35. C
36. C
37. B
38. D
39. A
40. C
41. D
42. A
43. B
44. B
45. D
46. D
47. C
48. D
49. C
50. D
51. A
52. B

Chapter 48—
Interstitial
Lung Disease
1. A
2. A
3. D
4. C
5. B
6. C
7. A
8. E
9. D
10. B
11. D
12. C
13. C
14. B
15. A
16. D
17. D
18. C
19. A
20. B
21. B

Chapter 49—
Pulmonary
Vascular Disease
1. B
2. D
3. D
4. D
5. A
6. E
7. B
8. C
9. A
10. D
11. C
12. A
13. C
14. B
15. C
16. A
17. C
18. B
19. A
20. D

Chapter 50—
Pneumonia
1. D
2. D
3. C
4. B
5. A

6. D
7. B
8. A
9. B
10. D
11. B
12. C
13. D
14. B
15. A
16. D
17. A
18. C
19. B
20. C
21. A
22. C
23. E
24. B
25. F
26. A
27. D
28. C
29. C
30. C
31. A
32. A

Chapter 51—
Cystic Fibrosis
1. A
2. C
3. D
4. B
5. A
6. D
7. B
8. C
9. D
10. A
11. E
12. F
13. C
14. B
15. D
16. B
17. A
18. C
19. C
20. B
21. E
22. D
23. A
24. B
25. C
26. D

Chapter 52—
Acute Respiratory
Distress Syndrome
1. A
2. D
3. B
4. A
5. B
6. A
7. A
8. B
9. C
10. C
11. A
12. D
13. D
14. C
15. D
16. B
17. D
18. C
19. A
20. B
21. D

Chapter 53—
Postoperative
Respiratory Care
1. D
2. D
3. A
4. C
5. D
6. C
7. B
8. A
9. C
10. B
11. B
12. C
13. A
14. B
15. A
16. D
17. B
18. A
19. C
20. D
21. D

Chapter 54—
Cardiac Failure
1. B
2. C
3. B
4. D

5. A
6. B
7. C
8. B
9. C
10. C
11. D
12. D
13. C
14. A
15. C
16. E
17. B
18. D
19. D
20. B
21. D
22. D
23. C
24. B
25. A
26. C
27. A
28. D
29. B
30. C
31. A
32. B
33. D
34. F
35. C
36. B
37. A
38. E
39. A
40. D
41. A
42. D
43. C
44. A
45. D
46. B
47. C
48. A
49. A
50. B
51. A

Chapter 55—
Chest Trauma
1. B
2. C
3. D
4. D
5. A
6. C

7. B
8. D
9. B
10. A
11. C
12. B
13. D
14. A
15. C
16. A
17. B
18. B
19. D
20. D
21. A

Chapter 56—Burn
and Inhalation Injuries
1. B
2. A
3. C
4. C
5. D
6. B
7. C
8. D
9. A
10. D
11. B
12. E
13. C
14. A
15. B
16. D
17. A
18. D
19. A
20. C

Chapter 57—
Neuromuscular
Dysfunction
1. D
2. B
3. D
4. C
5. A
6. D
7. B
8. C
9. D
10. A
11. C
12. A
13. B
14. D

15. D
16. A
17. C
18. C
19. D
20. A
21. B
22. C
23. A
24. B
25. C
26. A
27. B
28. C
29. D
30. B
31. B
32. B
33. A
34. B
35. C
36. D
37. A
38. C
39. B
40. A
41. D
42. C
43. A
44. D

Chapter 58—
Management of
Obstructive Sleep
Apnea Syndrome
1. B
2. D
3. B
4. C
5. A
6. D
7. C
8. A
9. B
10. C
11. A

Chapter 59—
Lung Cancer
1. D
2. B
3. C
4. D
5. A
6. D
7. C

8. E
9. A
10. B
11. C
12. D
13. B
14. A
15. E
16. C
17. D
18. B
19. C
20. D
21. A
22. B
23. A
24. B
25. C
26. A
27. D